Keto Diet for Beginners

A Step by Step Guide for Beginners to Ketogenic Diet and Lose Weight Fast with 120 Healthy Recipes

By Cameron Hamilton

Table of Contents

Chapter 5: Eating Keto on the Go 52

Chapter 6: Breakfast Recipes 62

Chapter 7: Lunch Recipes 80

Chapter 8: Dinner Recipes 94

Chapter 9: Snack Recipes 119

Chapter 10: Dessert Recipes 134

Conclusion 152

Introduction

Congratulations on downloading *Keto Diet for Beginners: Step by step guide for beginners to ketogenic diet and lose weight fast with 120 healthy recipes* and thank you for doing so. Making the decision to change your eating habits for the better is a big step and one that you should be applauded for making. It is also the easiest step, unfortunately, which is why this book is here to guide you through your transition to the ketogenic lifestyle. While it won't always be easy going, in the end, you will transform your body into a lean, mean, fat-burning machine.

To help you get started doing just that, the following chapters will discuss everything you need to know about the ketogenic diet and what makes it effective. This will start with an explanation of just what ketosis is, and why you want your body to attain this state as soon as possible. Next, you will learn about the macro and micronutrients that you are going to become very familiar within the coming weeks. Then you will learn about a wide variety of different tips that will not only help get you into ketosis as quickly as possible but ensure you remain there as well.

From there, you will learn all about how to get started on the keto diet successfully, and how to remain on the keto diet when you are out and about in the real world. You will then find plenty of different breakfast, lunch, dinner, snack, and dessert recipes to ensure you aren't lacking any healthy options while you adjust to your new lifestyle. Finally, you will find a 14-day meal plan that will get you through the keto transition period and see you come out the other side stronger than ever.

There are plenty of books on this subject on the market, thanks again for choosing this one! Every effort was made to ensure it is full of as much useful information as possible, please enjoy!

Chapter 1: Keto Diet Basics

If you don't consume enough carbs from your food, your cells will begin to burn fat for the necessary energy instead. Your body will switch over to ketosis for its energy source as you cut back on carbs and calories.

Two elements that occur when your body doesn't need the glucose:

- *The Stage of Lipogenesis:* If there is a sufficient supply of glycogen in your liver and muscles, any excess is converted to fat and stored.

- *The Stage of Glycogenesis*: The excess of glucose converts to glycogen and is stored in the muscles and liver. Research indicates that only about half of your energy used daily can be saved as glycogen.

Your body will have no more food (similar to when you are sleeping), making your body burn the fat to create ketones. Once the ketones break down the fats, which generate fatty acids, they will burn-off in the liver through beta-oxidation. Thus, when you no longer have a supply of glycogen or glucose, ketosis begins and will use the consumed/stored fat as energy.

Principles of the Keto Diet

The keto diet will set up your body to deplete the stored glucose. Once that is accomplished, your body will focus on diminishing the stored fat you have saved as fuel. Many people don't understand that counting calories don't matter at this point since it is just used as a baseline. Your body doesn't need glucose which will trigger these two stages:

- *The State of Glycogenesis*: The excess of glucose converts itself into glycogen, which is stored in the muscles and liver. Research indicates only about <u>half</u> of your energy used daily can be saved as glycogen.

- *The State of Lipogenesis:* This phase is introduced when there is an adequate supply of glycogen in your liver and muscles, with any excess being converted to fat and stored.

Your body will have no more food (similar to the times when you are sleeping), making your body burn the fat to create ketones. Once the ketones break down the fats, which generate fatty acids, they will burn-off in the liver through beta-oxidation. Thus, when you no longer have a supply of glycogen or glucose, ketosis begins and will use the consumed/stored fat as energy. When the glycerol and fatty acid molecules are released, the ketogenesis process begins, and acetoacetate is produced. The Acetoacetate is converted to two types of ketone units:

- *Acetone:* This is mostly excreted as waste but can also be metabolized into glucose. This is the reason individuals on a ketogenic diet will experience a distinctive smelly breath.

- *Beta-hydroxybutyrate or BHB:* Your muscles will convert the acetoacetate into BHB, which will fuel your brain after you have been on the keto diet for a short time.

How to Do It Right

You must decide how you want to proceed with your diet plan. It is always best to discuss this essential step with your physician. There are four methods, so you better understand the different levels of the keto diet plan. As a guideline use these standards to stay within your chosen carbohydrate limits on the keto plan:

- *Method # 1:* The standard ketogenic diet (SKD) is composed of moderate protein, high-fat, and is low in carbohydrates.

Typically, this phase of the diet is considered a high-fat (75%, low-carbohydrate (5%), and moderate protein (20%) diet plan. These are average counts and can vary.

- *Method # 2:* If you work out or are very active, you will call for the targeted keto diet, which is also called TKD. The process involves adding additional carbohydrates to the diet plan during the times when you're more active.

- *Method # 3:* The cyclical ketogenic diet (CKD) requires a restricted five-day keto diet plan followed by two high-carbohydrate days.

- *Method 4:* The high-protein keto diet is comparable to the standard keto plan (SKD) in all aspects. You will consume more protein. Its ratio is repeatedly noted as maintaining 35% protein, 5% carbs, and 60% fat. (Once again, these are average percentages.)

The Internet provides you with several ways to calculate your daily intake of carbs. Try an easy to follow <u>keto calculator</u> for assistance. Begin your weight loss process by making a habit of checking your levels when you want to know what essentials your body needs during the course of your dieting plan. You will document your personal information, such as height and weight. The Internet calculator will provide you with essential math.

Supplementation

The ketogenic diet has many benefits, but it's possible some of the essential nutrients are being overlooked in your menu planning. You may need to supplement to replace minerals, including magnesium, potassium, calcium, and sodium which comes from some of the food items not used on the keto diet. These electrolytes control muscle and nerve function and many other issues. Below are just a few of the ways you can supplement your plan:

- *Add Fish Oil To Your Diet:* Purchase this at any health food store in either the liquid or capsule form. The oil provides a natural anti-inflammatory content and also contributes to the higher fat intake requirements on the ketogenic diet.

- *Use MCT Oils:* Your ketogenic experience can improve with the use of MCT oil or medium-chain triglycerides. These fatty acids are found in its natural form in palm and coconut oil. Its advantages include the following:

    o The oil helps lower your blood sugar.

- o The use of MCTs makes it much easier to get into – and remain in ketosis. It is a natural anti-convulsive.

  - o It is also excellent for appetite control and weight loss.

- *Replace The Electrolytes:* If you have a low level of electrolytes, especially potassium and sodium, you can frequently suffer from fatigue, headaches, and constipation, which is commonly called keto flu. The low-carbs can also cause the kidneys to dump excess water, sodium and other valuable electrolytes that must be replenished.

- *Consume Plenty Of Sodium:* The amount of sodium required differs from other diet plans because other plans generally focus on less sodium. The sodium is lost with the water loss, so you will need to increase the sodium intake to keep the right balance of electrolytes. This is crucial, especially during the initial phase of the diet.

  - o Gain sodium in these ways:

    - Drinking bone broth regularly

- Adding salt to your food - Himalayan sea salt is a good choice.

  - Enjoy more sodium-rich foods including eggs and red meats

  - Be sure to monitor your blood pressure because sodium can have an effect on your pressure levels if you're are prone to hypertension.

- *Increase Magnesium Intake:* One of the most evident signs of a deficiency in magnesium is muscle cramps and fatigue. A blood test is the best way to test for possible problems. Magnesium has many benefits, including proper nerve and muscle function, helps maintain normal heart rhythm, assists over 300 body reactions including supporting adequate testosterone levels and working with calcium to keep your bones healthy.

  - Ideally, men should consume 420 mg. daily; women need only 320 mg. Eat some of these foods to maintain adequate magnesium levels:
    - Leafy green vegetables
    - Pumpkin seeds

- Avocados
- Almonds
- High-fat yogurts

- *Consume More Potassium:* Your normal blood pressure, regular heart rate, and fluid balance are aided by potassium. You need to remain cautious about adding potassium supplements to your diet because too much can cause an overload, which could be toxic.

  - Eat the following foods instead:
    - Salmon
    - Mushrooms
    - Avocados
    - Leafy greens
    - Nuts

Examples of What You Can Eat

Proteins

When looking for proteins to eat while on the ketogenic diet, you are going to want to focus on those that are grass-fed and pasture-raised. This, in turn, will help to ensure that your overall exposure to growth hormones and bacteria that are generated from unsafe farming practices remains at a minimum. As a general rule, you are going to want to stick with dark meat, and fatty fish as these will have more of the healthy fats your body will soon need. Roughly 25 percent of your diet should come from healthy proteins.

80/20 Ground beef (4 oz.)	280 calories	23g fat	0g net carbs	20g protein
Ribeye steak (4 oz.)	330 calories	25g fat	0g net carbs	27g protein
Beef Roast (4 oz.)	260 calories	20g fat	0g net carbs	19g protein
Beef pepperoni (5 slices)	110 calories	10g fat	0g net carbs	5g protein
Bacon (4 oz.)	519 calories	51g Fat	0g net carbs	13g protein
Porkchop (4 oz.)	286 calories	18g fat	0g net carbs	30g protein

Pork dust (.5 oz.)	80 calories	5g fat	0g net carbs	8g protein
Sausage (2 links)	120 calories	10g fat	0g net carbs	8g protein
Pork loin (3.5 oz.)	142 calories	4g fat	0g net carbs	26g protein
Chicken thigh (4 oz.)	250 calories	20g fat	0g net carbs	17g protein
Chicken breast (4 oz.)	125 calories	1g fat	0g net carbs	26g protein
Chicken wings (4 oz.)	250 calories	18g fat	0g net carbs	21g protein
Salmon (4 oz.)	236 calories	15g fat	0g net carbs	23g protein
Lobster (4 oz.)	114 calories	.68g fat	1g net carbs	24g protein
Sardines (1 can)	191 calories	11g fat	0g net carbs	23g protein
Tuna (1 packet)	70 calories	.5g fat	0g net carbs	17g protein
Ground lamb (4 oz.)	319 calories	27g fat	0g net carbs	19g protein
Liver (4 oz.)	135 calories	5g fat	0g net carbs	19g protein
Ground bison (4 oz.)	190 calories	11g fat	0g net carbs	23g protein
Deer (4 oz.)	130 calories	2g fat	0g net carbs	26g protein

Egg (1 large)	70 calories	5g fat	0.5g net carbs	6g protein
Almond butter (2 tbsp.)	180 calories	16g fat	4g net carbs	6g protein

Fats

As previously noted, fats should make up a majority of your diet while you are following a keto lifestyle. Many animal-based proteins are going to be naturally high in fat, as well. There are plenty of healthy, fatty oils to choose from. Just be sure to stay away from those that include trans fats.

Avocado (1)	322 calories	15g fat	2g net carbs	2g protein
Butter (1 T)	102 calories	12g fat	0g net carbs	0g protein
Coconut oil (1 T)	117 calories	14g fat	0g net carbs	0g protein
Olive oil (1 T)	119 calories	14g fat	0g net carbs	0g protein

Seeds and Nuts

Seeds and nuts are a useful way to add additional fat and protein to any meal. Some can be surprisingly high in carbohydrates, however, so it is important to be aware of the macros of the nuts you are considering before you add them to a meal lest you accidentally risk your ketogenic state without even realizing it.

Macadamia nuts (2 oz.)	407 calories	43g fat	3g net carbs	4g protein
Brazil nuts (2 oz.)	373 calories	37g fats	3g net carbs	8g protein
Pecans (2 oz.)	392 calories	41g fat	3g net carbs	5g protein
Almonds (2 oz.)	328 calories	28g fat	5g net carbs	12g protein
Hazelnuts (2 oz.)	356 calories	36g fat	3g net carbs	9g protein
Sunflower seeds (1T)	46 calories	4g fat	1g net carbs	1g protein
Flax seeds (1 T)	55 calories	4g fat	0g net carbs	2g protein
Hemp seeds (3 T)	170 calories	13g fat	0g net carbs	10g protein

Nut and Seed Butters and Flours

As traditional grain-based products are now off the table, you are going to likely find yourself turning to seed and nut-based substitutes on a regular basis. Seed and nut flours work just as well as traditional alternatives when it comes to desserts, and other baked goods and seed and nut butters often have higher overall fat contents than traditional butters.

Almond Butter (1 T)	98 calories	9g fat	1g net carbs	3g protein
Coconut butter (1 T)	117 calories	14g fat	0g net carbs	0g protein
Sunflower seed butter (1 T)	99 calories	9g fat	2g net carbs	3g protein
Tahini (1 T)	89 calories	8g fat	2g net carbs	3g protein
Almond Flour (2 oz.)	324 calories	28g fat	6g net carbs	12g protein
Coconut Flour (2 oz.)	120 calories	4g fat	6g net carbs	4g protein
Chia Seed Meal (2 oz.)	265 calories	17g fat	3g net carbs	8g protein
Flaxseed	224	18g	1g	8g

Meal (2 oz.)	calories	fat	net carbs	protein
Unsweetened Coconut (2 oz.)	445 calories	40g fat	8g net carbs	4g protein

<u>*Dairy Products*</u>

While admittedly not for everyone, dairy products are a great source for fat and a reasonable source of protein as well. Aim for organic and raw dairy products, if possible, as processed dairy tends to have a high carbohydrate count than non-processed dairy.

Heavy cream (1 oz.)	100 calories	12g fat	0g net carbs	0g protein
Greek yogurt (1 oz.)	28 calories	1g fat	1g net carbs	3g protein
Mayonnaise (1 oz.)	180 calories	20g fat	0g net carbs	0g protein
Half and Half (1 oz.)	40 calories	4g fat	1g net carbs	1g protein
Cottage cheese (1 oz.)	25 calories	1g fat	1g net carbs	4g protein
Cream Cheese (1 oz.)	94 calories	9g fat	1g net carbs	2g protein
Mascarpone (1 oz.)	120 calories	13g fat	0g net carbs	2g protein
Mozzarella (1 oz.)	70 calories	5g fat	1g net carbs	5g protein
Brie	95	8g	0g	6g

(1 oz.)	calories	fat	net carbs	protein
Aged Cheddar (1 oz.)	110 calories	9g fat	0g net carbs	7g protein
Parmesan (1 oz.)	110 calories	7g fat	1g net carbs	10g protein

Fruits and Vegetables

As a general rule, when following the ketogenic diet, you are going to want to severely limit the number of fruits that you eat as a vast majority are high in carbs. When it comes to vegetables, cruciferous, leafy green vegetables that grow above the ground are almost always a fine choice, while those that grow below ground should be consumed in moderation as they tend to have higher concentrations of carbohydrates.

Cabbage (6 oz.)	43 calories	0g fat	6g net carbs	2g protein
Cauliflower (6 oz.)	40 calories	0g fat	6g net carbs	5g protein
Broccoli (6 oz.)	58 calories	1g fat	7g net carbs	5g protein
Spinach (6 oz.)	24 calories	0g fat	1g net carbs	3g protein
Romaine Lettuce (6 oz.)	29 calories	1g fat	2g net carbs	2g protein
Green Bell Pepper (6 oz.)	33 calories	0g fat	5g net carbs	1g protein
Baby Bella Mushrooms (6 oz.)	40 calories	0g fat	4g net carbs	6g protein
Green Beans (6 oz.)	26 calories	0g fat	4g net	2g protein

			carbs	
Yellow Onion (6 oz.)	68 calories	0g fat	12g net carbs	2g protein
Blackberries (6 oz.)	73 calories	1g fat	8g net carbs	2g protein
Raspberries (6 oz.)	88 calories	1g fat	8g net carbs	2g protein

Carbohydrates

As previously noted, you may be able to add a small amount of carbs back into your diet without knocking yourself out of ketosis. Finding the right carbs to add back into your diet, however, as it doesn't take much of a given food to add up quickly. Keep the following list in mind when it comes to some of the most common carbs.

Sweet potatoes (1 small)	112 calories	0g fat	22g net carbs	2g protein
Acorn Squash (1 c)	56 calories	0g fat	13g net carbs	1g protein
Spaghetti squash (1 c)	42 calories	0g fat	8g net carbs	1g protein
Carrots (1 medium)	25 calories	0g fat	4g net carbs	0g protein
Peas (.5 c)	59 calories	0g fat	7g net carbs	4g protein
Cherries (1 c)	42 calories	.5g fat	16g net carbs	2g protein
Pears (1 medium)	65 calories	1g fat	7g net carbs	1.5g protein
Raspberries (1 c)	102 calories	0g fat	21g net carbs	.5g protein

Blackberries **(1 c)**	62 calories	1g fat	6g net carbs	2g protein
Watermelon **(1 wedge)**	87 calories	.5g fat	21g net carbs	2g protein

Chapter 2: Understanding Micro and Macronutrients

Fats

Even though plenty of research has been done to show that fat is not an evil thing. There are so many myths floating around about fat. I hope to debunk a few of those myths now.

Myth number one: "Fat has no nutrients." False. The truth is that fat is chock-full of nutrients. It is loaded with vitamins, and there are tons of benefits that come with fat that many people do not know about. Having a healthy consumption of healthy fats can help you maintain your goal weight by balancing your metabolism. Healthy fats can also help prevent depression since depression can sometimes be caused by a lack of cholesterol and fat in the brain. Fat can also stabilize your blood sugar level and results in a steady supply of energy.

Myth number two: "Fat makes you fat." Oh no, it does not. When excess carbohydrates need to be stored away in your body, your body converts them and creates body fat. Also, eating more dietary fat can actually help you to lose weight. Fat helps keep you full and reduces hunger pains, which result in less overeating and binging. Plus, omega-3 fatty acids activate the genes that help with fat burning and deactivate the genes that store fat. Not to mention that a healthy intake of fat can help balance your hormones, which makes losing and maintaining your weight much easier.

Myth number three: "Fat causes heart disease and clogs up your arteries." No, what clogs your arteries is cholesterol. Yes, cholesterol can be found in fat, but dietary cholesterol does not have much of an effect on the level of cholesterol in your blood. Further, increasing the intake of fat in your diet reduces the triglycerides floating in your blood. Since triglycerides are the main cause of heart disease, how can an increased consumption of dietary fat cause heart disease?

Saturated Fats

The key to having a healthy fat consumption is to minimize the consumption of food rich in saturated fats. Although your body needs both kinds of fat, saturated fats from foods derived from plants are enough to provide you with your saturated fat needs. Having high levels of saturated fat in your body leads to heart and cardiovascular disease.

Moreover, it is not enough to replace saturated fat-rich foods with fat-free food products as these are high in carbohydrates and increase the risk of the same disease mentioned. Take a look at the back of a fat-free product and a full-fat product like cream cheese. Notice that in the fat-free product, there is a lot more sugar than there is in the full-fat one. This is because manufacturers know fat equals flavor. When fat is removed from food, it winds up tasting terrible or is just plain tasteless. They want to make their money, so they add in sugar because they know that consumers love sugar. And what do we know sugar is converted to in your body? That's right, fat! So, you may think you are doing your body good by eating all the fat-free things on the market, but in actuality, you are feeding your body excess sugar, which is filling your body up with even more fat.

We know now that saturated fats are not anywhere near as bad as they were once touted to be. It was once feared that a diet heavy in saturated fat would raise cholesterol. Through studies over the years, it has been determined that it is actually a diet rich in carbohydrates that can increase coronary heart disease. This is because a diet high in carbohydrates lowers HDL cholesterol and increases the small particle LDL cholesterol. It is not the saturated fat or the cholesterol from dietary sources that raise the level of the small bad LDL cholesterol. It is the consumption of too many carbohydrates. Saturated fat is actually great for your liver, your brain, your heart, your nervous system, and more.

Other health benefits to regularly consuming saturated fat include boosting your metabolism, immune system strengthening, reversing inflammatory disease, helps your body more effectively process calcium, and is a wonderful carrier for fat-soluble vitamins.

Chicken, lamb, beef, butter, bacon, and coconut oil are all good sources of healthy saturated fats.

Monounsaturated Fats

Monounsaturated fats come mostly from oils and nuts. Monounsaturated fats are another kind of fat that you can consume often without too much worry. They provide several health benefits, especially when you use them instead of trans fats. Make sure that the oils you are using are processed minimally. The words to look for are "expeller pressed", "cold-pressed", or "centrifuge extracted". When using these oils, there is not a large chance of intaking oxidized fats. This is good because oxidized fats can cause damage to your cells.

Why you should exercise caution when consuming monounsaturated fats, there are some great health benefits. Monounsaturated fats can help reduce belly fat when your intake of carbs is also reduced, these fats can decrease your risk of breast cancer, and they can also encourage weight loss when used instead of trans fats.

Avocados, olive oil, almond oil, avocado oil, macadamia nuts, and hazelnuts are good sources of monounsaturated fats.

Polyunsaturated Fats

Polyunsaturated fats should be used very sparingly. They are quite likely to oxidize during heating, so they are not good for cooking. Remember that when fats are oxidized, they can cause damage to your cells. There are some polyunsaturated fats that are not terrible. They are actually considered essential fatty acids for your body's functioning. Omega-3 and omega-6 are two of these. Your body is unable to produce these fatty acids itself, but they are must for your body to be able to function properly. They must be received through food. However, too much omega-6 can cause an increase in inflammatory diseases like autoimmune disorders, irritable bowel syndrome, arthritis, cancer, and metabolic syndrome.

You must be very careful when eating foods that contain polyunsaturated fats. Do not eat them very often. That being said, there are health benefits to eating polyunsaturated fats. Consuming omega-6s is wonderful for brain and muscle development. They also add support to your nervous system; your immune system and they are great for helping your brain and body communicate through hormones. The consumption of omega-3 fatty acids can help improve bone strength and can help reduce inflammatory substances in your body. Having a good ratio of omega 6's and omega 3's is optimal for your health.

Some good sources of omega-3 and omega-6 essential fatty acids are foods that contain healthy levels of polyunsaturated fats. Good options for these are salmon, trout, flax seeds, hemp seeds, and chia seeds. Make sure that these are not heated very high so that they do not oxidize.

Trans Fats

Trans fats should be avoided at all costs. Very minimal amounts of trans fats are created in nature. You will find tiny amounts of dairy and meat, and these natural trans fats can actually be beneficial. However, most trans fats are made in factories. These are "hydrogenated fats", and are made when hydrogen is added to fats to make them solid at room temperature. Making the fats solidify at room temperature has the added effect of ensuring food will have a longer shelf life. This benefit is only for the manufacturers, not your body's cells. Trans fats are known to be harmful to your health in many ways. Increasing your risk of type 2 diabetes, contributing to heart disease, damaging your memory, and highly increasing inflammation in your body are just a few of the health problems caused by the consumption of trans fats.

There are really no good reasons to consume trans fats. You should absolutely avoid them

Manufactured trans fats are found in products such as:
- Baked goods like cake, pie crusts, and crackers, and ready-made frosting
- Snacks like packaged microwave popcorn, and potato, corn, and tortilla chips.
- Fried food due to the oil used in the cooking process
- Refrigerator dough like canned biscuits, cinnamon rolls, and frozen pizza crusts
- Non-dairy coffee creamer
- Margarine
- In food labels, trans fat can also be listed as shortening, hydrogenated oil, partially hydrogenated oil, and hydrogenated vegetable oil.

If you pick up a package of food and it has trans fats listed in the ingredients section, put it down and run far, far away.

Protein

Most foods, including vegetables and grains, contain some amount of protein. You would be surprised at how much of a protein powerhouse a serving of normal green peas can be! Foods that have substantial amounts of protein are meat from animals, dairy products, beans, and nuts. Protein can provide energy for your body; however, being a source of energy is not the primary purpose of protein.

You read earlier that your body takes the proteins you feed it and breaks them down into amino acids. When the protein is broken down into amino acids, the body then uses them to create its own proteins intended for various purposes. With the 20 amino acids that your body would need, it can create an infinite number of proteins like enzymes for chemical reactions, hormones for triggering organs, collagen for bone structure, and antibodies for the immune system.

Your body's proteins are constantly broken down and re-synthesized to build more proteins. Most of the amino acids from broken down protein are reused, but some are lost and must be replaced through your diet.

Protein serves many purposes in your body. Protein can reduce cravings, it can lower the hunger hormone ghrelin, it can benefit your bone health and workout recovery, it lowers your triglycerides comment and increases fat burning, it can provide balanced ratios of vitamins minerals and fatty acids, and it is the building block for muscle repair and growth.

While protein does have many benefits, it can be kind of a double-edged sword. If you remember, we talked about gluconeogenesis before, which is when the excess protein you eat is converted into glucose and then stored as fat in your body. If you are eating too much protein, then your body will take the converted glucose from it and use it as fuel rather than the ketones you want your body to use as fuel. On the flip side, you have to eat enough protein, or your body will start to use your muscles for fuel.

In following a ketogenic diet, you are taking the carbohydrates away from your body, drastically reducing your glucose levels. Remember, there are certain parts of the body that can run only on glucose, like your red blood cells and parts of your brain. Your body will still need to find sources of glucose to perform these functions. When in ketosis, the best way for your body to source glucose will be from the protein you eat. Gluconeogenesis will not just randomly start eating away at the protein in your muscles for glucose unless it has no other source for it. If you eat too little protein, your muscles will be gobbled up by your body so that your brain and red blood cells can function properly.

It is a really delicate balance to ensure you have enough protein to make sure your body does not eat your muscles, but not so much that your body starts converting the protein into glucose and storing it away as fat.

One common artificial sweetener is Sucralose, better known as Splenda. Many people think they are making a better choice by using Splenda because they believe that it is free of calories. Because sucralose is 600 times sweeter than sugar when used in its pure liquid form, only a small amount of it is needed to sweeten the foods it is in. However, to replace granulated sugar in baked goods and other things, the manufacturers of Splenda bulk it up with other sweeteners. It is bulked up with dextrose and maltodextrin, which are undesirable sweeteners that are not free of calories. There are 96 calories and 32 grams of carbohydrates in just one cup of Splenda. Most people think Splenda is a great, calorie-free alternative to processed sugar. This is dangerous, especially for diabetics! Splenda has also been proven to have a negative effect on the functioning of your thyroid, and it makes it hard for your body to absorb zinc and iodine. It can also make an irritable bowel syndrome worse because it lowers the number of good bacteria in your gut.

For the sake of your health, just avoid all artificial sweeteners. Anything that ends in "ose" (dextrose, fructose, sucralose, etc.) is a form of sugar that you do not want in your body.

There are better, more natural sweeteners to choose from. Even so, some of these options are obviously better than others. Some of the less desirable options are:

Honey is far less refined than table sugar; however, it is still really high in calories and fructose. In a single teaspoon of honey, there are 22 calories. That is actually more calories than you would get in the same measurement of sugar (1 tsp = 15 calories). The main issue with honey is that it is almost 50% fructose. Honey is more nutritious than table sugar in that it contains vitamins and minerals that are necessary for your body, but it only contains tiny traces of them. Honey is not a healthy alternative to sugar regardless of these vitamins and minerals. You should use it very sparingly, if at all. Your body does not know if you are feeding it table sugar or honey. Once it is in your bloodstream, sugar is sugar and will be processed as such.

Agave is marketed as a health food. It is touted by its manufacturers as a better option for diabetics since it has a small effect on the blood sugar, and it is all-natural. Just because it is sold in the health food aisle does not make it healthy. Processed sugar Is about 50% fructose, but agave is almost 90% fructose. It is absolutely not a better option than regular table sugar.

Coconut sugar is said to be lower on the glycemic index than regular sugar, and more nutrition. Coconut sugar also contains a fiber called inulin. Scientists think that inulin helps to slow the rate at which your body absorbs glucose. There are not very many nutrients in coconut sugar, and it has the same number of non-nutritive calories as regular sugar. Even though you may see claims that coconut sugar is fructose free, this is misleading. It is up to 80% sucrose. Sucrose is actually made up of half glucose and half fructose. Basically, coconut sugar gives your body just as much glucose as regular sugar. It is also not a good option for sweetener when you are trying to kick it into ketosis.

Food manufacturers have gotten wise to the fact that consumers are paying more attention to the ingredients in the food they are selling. Because of this, you have to do some sleuthing when purchasing food. You will need to read all the labels on the food products you buy to ensure you are not getting hidden sweeteners. What can be even more frustrating is that as soon as you seem to get used to a specific sweetener being used in a certain food product, the food companies change it upon you. Some of the sweeteners you need to look out for are beet sugar, cane crystals, fruit juice concentrate, corn syrup solids, palm sugar, turbinado sugar, brown rice syrup, sorghum syrup, etc. There are so many to look out for, and it can be really frustrating. Sometimes it is just easier to stick with the products that contain sweeteners you know are safe.

Some of the better options for sugar alternatives are Stevia, erythritol, xylitol, and monk fruit.

You can even purchase blends of some of these that have been formulated to mimic processed sugar as closely as possible without the glucose spike. What exactly are these alternative sweeteners, though?

Stevia is a plant-based sweetener made from the leaves of the Stevia plant. Stevia is a very concentrated sweetener that is around 200 to 300 times sweeter than sugar. Because of this, a very little goes a very long way making Stevia an economical choice for sweetening your foods. Stevia is truly calorie-free and has no carbohydrates, either. You will probably notice that your local grocery store sells products that claim to be Stevia. Be careful with these, and read the labels. Too many of these products are cut with other sweeteners like dextrose or maltodextrin to bulk them up and make them go further. Look for pure Stevia. You are more likely to find pure Stevia in a store that sells healthier options, like Whole Foods or Sprout than in Wal-Mart or Piggly Wiggly.

Stevia glycerite is another form of Stevia. It is more of a syrup consistency. Sometimes the powdered Stevia can have a bitter aftertaste, but this is not the case with the Stevia Glycerite. The glycerite is still hundreds of times sweeter than sugar, and a little goes a long way.

Monk fruit is derived from a plant that grows in the mountains in China. It is also known as Lo

Han Kuo. Similar to Stevia, it is around 300 times sweeter than sugar. You can purchase monk fruit in powdered or liquid form. Again, be on the lookout for sweeteners you want to avoid, like dextrose and maltodextrin. You can sometimes find monk fruit blended with erythritol, which is a safe alternative sweetener choice.

Erythritol is a sweetener that can be made from corn or birch. Birch is the better option, as corn can be heavily GMO. Erythritol can be found in the granular or powdered form. It is not known for causing stomach distress as some other sweeteners can, and it too is zero calories and has no effect on your blood sugar. Your body does actually process and absorbs erythritol, but it is generally all used up long before it gets to your colon. For some people, erythritol can cause a strange cooling sensation in the mouth, but this does not happen to everyone and is not harmful.

Xylitol is another great choice for an alternative sweetener. While it has a few calories, and will ever so slightly affect your blood sugar, it is minimal and far better than processed sugar. Xylitol is probably the closest you will get to have the taste and texture of processed sugar. Xylitol is also good for your teeth. Some downsides of xylitol are that is can definitely cause a stomach upset if you eat too much of it. Also, it is very dangerous for dogs. Even a small amount can cause major health problems or death. So, if you have a fur baby, xylitol is not the sweetener for you.

There are also a few blends of alternative sweeteners that you can purchase in-store or online. Pyure is a blend of erythritol and Stevia. You can find it in granulated form. Just be sure you do not buy the one that has sugar in it for bulk. It has no calories or carbs and has no effect on your blood sugar. Swerve is a blend of erythritol and oligosaccharides (another form of sweetener that is safe to use). Swerve has no calories and no impact on your blood sugar levels. You can get swerve in granulated or powdered form, and it measures just like sugar, which is fantastic if you are a baker! I have seen both of these at Whole Foods, and I have seen Pyure at Wal-Mart and other local stores. You can also purchase them online.

Chapter 3: Beating the Keto Flu

After you have decided to go all-in on the keto diet, the first thing you are going to need to do is to prepare yourself for the hardships that are to come. Preparing yourself mentally for the challenge is a large part of making it through to the other side successfully. This means planning ahead and ensuring that you have as little extraneous activity going on during this week as possible. If you can, treat it as if you are going to be down sick for a week with the flu and plan accordingly. While this won't make it easier to make the transition less painful per se, it will make it easier to stay on track as you won't have as many distractions driving you back into the waiting arms of carbs of all shapes and sizes.

When it comes to cutting out carbs, some people's bodies are going to need a bit more help making it to the other side than others. If you are testing your acetone level (and you should be) and you find that you are having a hard time making it past the .5 market, then you will need to consider how much protein you are currently consuming. If you consume too much protein then it will turn in to glucose, causing the same issues that you would find if you just went ahead and kept eating carbs. becomes glucose, which raises your insulin levels, just like glucose created from carbs. If you can't seem to cut out the extra protein, add in more fat to balance things out. Start by adding a tablespoon of coconut oil and a tablespoon of melted butter to your morning coffee or tea and go from there. This will also allow you to start your day off feeling fuller in the morning which will help you to naturally shy away for extra carbs as well.

Testing Your Ketone Level

You must first determine that your body can undergo the diet and the massive adjustments it will be made to adapt to a fat-burning state. You must also determine your body fat percentage, weight, and other relevant data to create your personal macronutrient mix via keto calculators available online or the formulas provided to you earlier in the book.

I also urge you to consult with your doctor or healthcare provider before you begin, especially if you have any health problems. If you go to the doctor for no other reason, go to get your bloodwork done. It will be amazing to get your tests redone in a year and be able to see all the amazing changes that have been happening inside your body while the outside has been transforming as well.

Eat Better

While fully transitioning into the keto diet will help to ensure that you feel less full, overall, this change won't happen overnight. Until you find the right mix of macronutrients for your body, you may find yourself regularly feeling hungrier than before. While this is the case, it is important to make a conscious effort to eat full meals, as opposed to grazing on snacks, even keto-approved snacks, as this is a great way to stall the initial onslaught of weight loss that typically comes with the ketogenic transition. While a fat bomb or two per day is fine, they can add up quickly if you aren't paying attention, depriving you of the results of all of your hard work in the process.

When it comes to refilling your pantry with keto-approved items, it is important to stick with all-natural items in addition to those that are simply low in carbohydrates as the more processed an item is, the less room that is going to be left for nutritional value. However, it is not enough to simply look for items that are marked as low-carb, as this has become a marking phrase in line with no sugar added and fat-free, which may more may not have any actual bearing on the nutritional content of the item in question.

On the contrary, items that are truly healthy don't need to advertise this fact. The fat to carb ratio of an avocado isn't subject to debate, which means you never have to worry if it is actually as healthy as the label says. Avoid hype when it comes to what you put into your body, seek out organic, natural foods as much as possible.

Exercise More

When you are in the middle of the keto flu, one of the last things you are going to want to do is to exercise, much less exercise vigorously. Unfortunately, studies show that this is exactly what you are going to want to do if you want your body to reach a ketogenic state as quickly as possible. Sticking with high intensity, cardio exercises will help your body burn through its reserves of glucose as quickly as possible, which means it will have no choice but to get its act together and start producing ketones to ensure it can continue functioning properly.

What follows is a variable list of exercises designed to force your body into a ketogenic state as quickly as possible. Your goal should be to undertake the most strenuous of the exercises that you can without causing yourself to feel dizzy or as though you may faint. Keep in mind that you are working on far less fuel than normal at this point and be sure not to overdo it.

- *10-minute-high intensity workout:* You will want to complete the entire circuit three times and take a 10-second rest between each set. Each circuit should take 3 minutes and 10 seconds.

- *Sumo squats:* Start with your feet at slightly more than hip-width apart and keep your toes pointed facing outward at a 45-degree angle. Place all of your weight on the heels of your feet, your chest upright, and your back straight. Lower yourself down towards the ground until your thighs are essentially parallel to the ground. Using your quads and your glutes, push yourself back into the starting position. To end each set, move into a reverse lung and fold your body forward while keeping your arms stretched overhead.

- *Jumping jacks:* Start by standing in a relaxed stance, with your feet about hip-width apart and your arms resting at your sides. Jump up while spreading your feet and raising your arms above your head. Repeat as many times as possible, as quickly as possible, for about 45 seconds. If keeping this up for the full length of time proves untenable, get your body used to the exercise by following through with the movement and leaving out the jumping.

- *Jab, cross, front kick (left):* Start with your left foot in front of your right foot and your hips facing right. Raise your arms so that you are in somewhat of a boxer stance. Start with a jab by punching forward with your left arm straight out. Move directly into throwing a cross by punching with your left arm and rotating your body to the right. This should leave the full weight of your body on your right foot, and your right heel should raise slightly off of the floor. End the sequence by kicking forward with your back foot.

- *Jab, cross-front kick (right):* The same as above but in reverse.

- *20-minute-high intensity workout*
- You will want to complete the entire circuit three times and take a 15-second rest between each set.

- *Side lunges:* Stand with the full weight of your body on your heels with your toes facing straight ahead. Take a wide step to the left so that you move into a full lunge, taking care to keep your knee straight above your toes. Return to the starting position and repeat with your other leg.

- *Triceps dips:* Start by sitting in a firm chair with your legs straight out in front of you. Using the seat of a chair for support, lower yourself off of it using your arms, one on either side of your waist. Lower yourself as close to the ground as possible before raising yourself all the way back up. Repeat as many times as possible.

- *Butt kickers:* Jog in place, extending your leg at the back of your stride so that your heel strikes your butt.

- *Squats:* Start in a relaxed position with your feet directly beneath your hips. Raise your hands, so they are parallel to the floor and slowly lower yourself towards the floor as far as possible before returning to the starting position. Repeat as many times as possible.

- *Pushups:* Begin this exercise by placing your hands on the ground at a width that is slightly wider than your shoulders while letting your weight rest on your hands and toes before lowering yourself to the ground and returning to the starting position after your chest almost touches the floor.

- *30-minute-high intensity workout*
  - You will want to complete the entire circuit three times and take a 15-second rest between each set.
    - Sit-ups
    - Jumping jacks
    - Side lunges
    - Triceps dips
    - Butt kickers

- Squats
- Push-ups

Stick with It

Once your body settles into a state of ketosis, you will likely notice a visible uptick in your overall weight loss, possibly even exceeding one pound per week. However, once you start getting closer to your weight loss goal, it is common for weight loss to drop to the pound a week mark. In fact, if you are looking to lose weight in the long-term, then about a pound per week is considered the healthy maximum. Eventually, your weight loss will slow even more, but this is only a sign that you are getting closer to your ideal weight.

Finally, it is important to be aware of the fact that everyone hits weight loss plateaus from time to time, and the only way to get through them is to stay the course. When you find yourself on a plateau, the worst thing you can do is try and switch up your entire weight loss routine, as this will just confuse your body even more and make it even more difficult for you to get your weight loss back in gear.

Chapter 5: Eating Keto on the Go

In reading this book and learning the methods you will need to follow to achieve ketosis through a ketogenic diet, you may be thinking that you will never leave the kitchen or grocery store again. That you will have to cook every single thing from scratch and will be spending the rest of your life reading every label in the store. While it is always best to cook for yourself (mostly because you know exactly what is in your food, plus it can be quite enjoyable), that is not always an option in the fast-paced lifestyle of the world we live in. You do not want to become an antisocial hermit just because you are trying to get healthy. In fact, our brains crave social interaction, so it would be crazy to shut yourself away from the life you are used to living. And yes, you will need to be vigilant in reading the labels on all the food you eat, especially in the first few months while you are getting accustomed to this way of eating. This will not be a forever thing though. Eventually, you will know what is keto-friendly and what is not. I would suggest periodically checking labels, though, as you never know when a food manufacturer will cut costs by switching from a keto-friendly ingredient to one you do not want to consume.

You absolutely can still go out to dinner with your spouse on a special night or to brunch with your parents on a Sunday afternoon, and you can still meet your friends for coffee after work during the week. Your life is not over because you are suddenly aware of all the bad foods out there. You still have wonderful and delicious options. You just have to know what is available, and not be afraid to ask questions or make special requests. Many people these days have allergies or special dietary needs, and most food places are more than happy to oblige their customers. You can still pop into the gas station on a road trip and feel good about the snacks you grab to munch on. And as for some of the special ingredients you may wish to keep on hand, many companies have begun to make them in individual packets making it easy to keep in your purse or gym bag for when you are on the go.

Snacks

When you are on the run, it is good to keep some non-perishable snacks with you. This way, no matter what your adventure brings, you will have something to eat. Good options are:

- Mixed nuts (single-serve packs or dish them into baggies, so you do not overdo it)
- Nut/seed butter (these can be found in individual packets in many stores now)

- Packets of salmon or tuna (they might stink up the car, but they will fuel you)
- Flax crackers (I have seen these in stores, but they are easy to make, too)
- Jerky (watch out for sugars. EPIC brand is a safe bet)
- Pork rinds (these may take some getting used to, but the crunch is very satisfying!)
- Seaweed crackers (find in the aisle of your store where they sell Asian foods.)
- Pickles (you can find single-serve ones in gas stations, but look out for sugar!)

If you are able to keep a small cooler, here are some other good snack ideas:

- Celery sticks with nut butter or cream cheese
- Cheese sticks
- Deli meat and cheese roll-ups
- Cooked bacon
- Guacamole
- Veggies that travel well, like cucumbers or zucchini

Restaurants

When eating out at restaurants, you may feel like your options are limited at first. I am here to tell you that this is not the case. You have just got to be brave and ask questions of the server, and do not be afraid to ask for substitutions if needed. No one will judge you if you ask for extra vegetables in place of the rice that is typically served with a dish.

- If you are eating in an Asian food restaurant, it can be a little tricky. Pretty much everything is covered in sauce and will have sugar. If it is a place where you can order rather than a buffet, ask for a serving of meat with no sauce, and a salad.

- In a restaurant serving Italian dishes, you might be hard-pressed to find keto-friendly options. Ask if you can substitute vegetables for your pasta, maybe having chicken alfredo over broccoli. Be sure to inquire how the alfredo is thickened, and if there is any flour. Chicken Marsala should be a safe option, as long as it is not dredged in flour before being cooked.

- Indian food is delicious, but you have to be vigilant here as well. Avoid vegetable curries since these are generally full of ingredients that will kick you out of ketosis. Also, be sure to ask which of the curries have been thickened with flour, and avoid those. Instead of bread or rice, go with some fresh vegetables. Opt for chicken shorba or chicken korma as your main dish.

- Tapas bars are usually a great option because you can typically get a plate with nothing but meats and vegetables. Just avoid the dishes that are bread-based.

- Mexican restaurants can be fairly easy, surprisingly! Choose a taco salad or ask for a burrito with no tortilla. They might give you funny looks, but you will enjoy your food with no ketosis problems.

- Sushi can be another tricky one. Obviously, you cannot have traditional sushi with its sticky white rice. Instead, go for sashimi dishes, with just the raw fish. They can be quite tasty and filling.

- For a pizza restaurant, just scrape the toppings off your serving of pizza. You can just eat the cheese, meat, and vegetables off of your plate with a fork or place them over a big salad. Try not to get too much of the sauce since most pizza sauce is loaded with sugar.

- When going somewhere like Denny's, Waffle House or IHOP, where breakfast can be ordered all day; you have good options, but still need to be careful. While an omelet is a great choice, usually, some of these places add pancake batter to them to make them fluffier. Just specify to your server that your omelet is to be made with real eggs, not their omelet batter. Most of these places offer lunch and dinner plates as well. Just look over the menu and choose options with plenty of meat and vegetables. Avoid ketosis killers, and you will be fine.

For the most part, just avoid the potatoes, rice, bread, noodles, fries; and be on the lookout for unwanted starches. Stick with meats and vegetables, and you will be good to go!

Fast Food

As far as fast food goes, these options can be super easy. Just be mindful of ingredients, condiments, and skip the bread and fries.

- Burger King and McDonald's both have food that you can easily customize to be keto-friendly. If it is breakfast time, just order one of their breakfast sandwiches and request no biscuit/muffin/etc. You can also order just a side or two of meat, and a couple sides of eggs. Easy-peasy. If it is lunch or dinner time, opt for a burger with no bun. The restaurant will usually serve it to you in a bowl and give you a fork. Just be sure to ask for no ketchup since that will be full of sugar. Instead of french fries, have a salad; and drink water instead of soda.

- Hardees/Carl's Jr is awesome, as they have keto-friendly meals already on the menu. If it is breakfast time, order their low-carb breakfast bowl, which will be filled with eggs, meats, and cheese. For lunch or dinner, you can order the lettuce-wrapped burger or a grilled chicken breast.

- Wendy's is a little trickier, as they do not offer much in the way of keto-friendly food. Avoid the salads at Wendy's as they are ridiculously high in carbs and will definitely knock you out of ketosis. Again, you can order a burger with no bun (baconator is great!) or a grilled chicken sandwich with no bun. Avoid carby sides like fries and opt for water instead of soda.

- Red Robin has a variety of options. You can get just about anything wrapped in lettuce, so just ask. When choosing your meal, be mindful of the sauces and toppings because many of them will be laden with sugar. Not a good thing. Also, ask for vegetables or a salad in place of the bottomless fries.

- If you are lucky enough to live by In-n-Out Burger, march right in there and order yourself something "protein style". I hear they also have a menu with just low carb options. It does not hurt to ask!

- Five Guys Burgers is one place that everyone should go when following a ketogenic diet. They do not even flinch when you ask for no bun; they just wrap it up in lettuce or serve it in a special bowl. At Five Guys, you can choose from a myriad of options off their board, adding pretty much anything you can dream of to your burger. They are a fantastic option and always delicious.

- Sandwich places like Jersey Mike's, Subway, Firehouse Subs, and Jimmy John's are surprisingly good options. You would not think so, being that they are sandwich shops, but most of them will make your food without bread or a wrap. At Subway, you can order any sandwich as a salad. Just be mindful of sugary sauces and dressings. At Jersey Mike's, you can order a "Sub in a Tub", and they will make your sandwich in a bowl. My favorite is Jimmy John's Unwich. They make any sandwich you want and wrap it snugly inside lettuce leaves. At these places, avoid the chips and soda.

- Chipotle. Moe's, Qdoba, and other Mexican chains can give you decent options as well. Most of these types of places will let you build your own burrito, and you can opt to do it as a burrito bowl instead of avoiding the tortilla. You can also go for a salad bowl with all sorts of toppings. Just avoid the rice and beans, and be careful when you start to pile on the toppings as the carbs can quickly add up, knocking you off the ketosis wagon.

- Chick-fil-a really does not boast much of a selection, unfortunately. Their grilled nuggets and grilled market salad are good, though.

- Popeyes is another place with little in the way of options. Your best bet is an order of their blackened tenders.

See, you do not have to hide at home now that you have taken your health into your own hands. It might be easier to do so the first few weeks while you are getting the hang of this new lifestyle, but it should not be permanent. There are plenty of foods you can enjoy while being social, and you can make sure that you remain in ketosis while doing so.

Chapter 6: Breakfast Recipes

Keto 90-Second French Toast

Yields Provided: 2 Servings
Macro Counts For Each Serving:
- Fat Content: 30 g
- Total Net Carbs: 4 g
- Protein: 12 g
- Calories: 352

What to Use
- Coconut flour (1 tbsp.)
- Melted butter (1.25 tbsp.)
- Egg (1)
- Cream cheese (1 tsp.)
- Bak. powder (.25 tsp.)
- Nutmeg (1 pinch)
- Cinnamon (.25 tsp.)

The Toast
- Egg (1)
- Heavy whipping cream (.25 cup)
- Lakanto Monkfruit Powdered Sugar (.25 tsp.)
- _Optional_: Sugar-Free Maple Syrup

What to Do
1. Melt butter in a glass bowl (6-inch).

2. Work in the remainder of the fixings, whisking until combined.
3. Cook for 1.5 minutes in the microwave.
4. Transfer to the countertop to cool for a minute or two. Cut the bread in half.
5. In a flat dish, whisk one egg and 1/4 cup of the heavy whipping cream.
6. Soak both sides of bread in egg/whipping cream mixture.
7. Heat one tablespoon of butter in a skillet and fry each side until crispy.
8. Sprinkle 1/4 teaspoon of the Swerve Confectioners' Sugar and serve with sugar-free syrup. Berries are also delicious.

Egg and Bacon Avocado

Yields Provided: 2 Servings
Macro Counts For Each Serving:
- Protein: 12 grams
- Net Carbs: 5.2 grams
- Fats: 26.2 grams
- Calories: 301

What to Use
- Salt (as desired)
- Pepper (as desired)
- Cheddar cheese (1 T shredded)
- Bacon (1 slice)
- Eggs (2)
- Avocado (1)

What to Do
1. Start by making sure your oven is heated to 425F.
2. Add the oil to a pan before placing the pan on the stove over a burner turned to a high/medium heat and let it melt before adding in the bacon and allowing it to fry until crispy before adding in the spinach.
3. Slice the avocado lengthwise before removing the pit and the skin and place both halves into a muffin tin to steady them while they cook.
4. Add half of the ingredients to each of the avocado halves, starting with the egg.
5. Place the muffin tin in the oven and let it cook for approximately 15 minutes.

6. Serve hot.

Avocado and Sausage Breakfast Sandwich

Yields Provided: 1 Serving
Macro Counts For Each Serving:
- Protein: 15 grams
- Net Carbs: 1.3 grams
- Fats: 26.4 grams
- Calories: 333

What to Use
- Salt (as desired)
- Pepper (as desired)
- Coconut oil (2 T)
- Avocado (.25 sliced)
- Sharp cheddar cheese (2 T)
- Cream cheese (1 T)
- Egg (1)
- Sausage patties (2)

What to Do
1. Add the oil to a pan before placing the pan on the stove over a burner turned to a high/medium heat. Add in the sausage and let it cook approximately 1 minute per side. Remove the sausage and retain the grease.
2. Add the cheeses to a small microwave-safe bowl before placing the bowel in the microwave for 30 seconds. Mix well.
3. Add the eggs to the pan and allow them to cook until they are firm on the bottom but still somewhat raw on top.

4. Add in the rest of the ingredients before using a spatula to fold the omelet in half. You will know it is finished cooking when it is a golden-brown color on the bottom.
5. Place the omelet on top of one piece of sausage and use the other to form a sandwich.

Egg Fast Cloud Bread

Yields Provided: 1 Serving
Macro Counts For Each Serving:
- Fat Content: 7.4 g
- Total Net Carbs: 0.6 g
- Protein: 4.2 g
- Calories: 85

What to Use
- Softened cream cheese (3 oz.)
- Large eggs (3)
- Salt (1 dash)
- _Optional:_ Cream of tartar preferred (1 pinch)

What to Do
1. Set the oven temperature at 300° Fahrenheit.
2. Prepare the baking pan.
3. Separate the eggs into another container.
4. Use an electric mixer to prepare the cream cheese with the salt. Add to the yolk - mixing well.
5. Whisk the cream of tartar in with the egg whites using clean mixer tongs.
6. Fold the egg yolks into the white mixture.
7. Scoop six portions onto the pan. Flatten slightly with a spatula.
8. Bake for about 24 to 30 minutes.
9. Let the loaf of bread cool in the baking pan for three to five minutes before moving to a cooling rack.

10. Freeze for better results or place in a
    zipper-type baggie in the fridge.

Mushroom Omelet

Yields Provided: 1 Serving
Macro Counts For Each Serving:
- Protein: 21 grams
- Net Carbs: 4 grams
- Fats: 34.6 grams
- Calories: 401

What to Use
- Salt (as desired)
- Pepper (as desired)
- Coconut oil (2 T)
- Mushrooms (3)
- Yellow onion (.25)
- Cheddar cheese (1 oz. shredded)
- Eggs (3)

What to Do
1. Add the eggs to a mixing bowl before seasoning and desired and whisking until the eggs are frothy.
2. Add the oil to a pan before placing the pan on the stove over a burner turned to medium heat. Add in the eggs and allow them to cook until they are firm on the bottom but still somewhat raw on top.
3. Add in the rest of the ingredients before using a spatula to fold the omelet in half. You will know it is finished cooking when it is a golden-brown color on the bottom.

Low-Carb Zucchini Walnut Bread

Yields Provided: 8 Servings
Macro Counts For Each Serving:
- Fat Content: 36 g
- Total Net Carbs: 6 g
- Protein: 10 g
- Calories: 397

What to Use
- Truvia or your favorite sweetener (.5 cup)
- Eggs (3)
- Ghee or Oil (.5 cup)
- Almond flour (1.5 cups)
- Bak. powder (1 tsp.)
- Coconut flour (.5 cup)
- Bak. soda (1 tsp.)
- Nutmeg (.25 tsp.)
- Cinnamon (.5 tsp.)
- Unsweetened almond milk (.5 cup)
- Chopped walnuts (1 cup)
- Shredded zucchini (2 cups)
- *Also Needed*: 6-cup bundt pan

What to Do
1. Set the oven at 350° Fahrenheit.
2. Grease the pan and set aside.
3. Toss the eggs, sweetener, and oil into the stand mixer mixing bowl. Use the paddle attachment to beat for 2 to 3 minutes until well incorporated.
4. Add the coconut and almond flour, baking powder, nutmeg, baking soda, cinnamon,

and almond milk. Continue mixing for
another two to three minutes.
5. Stir in the shredded zucchini and chopped
walnuts and arrange in the greased pan.
6. Bake for 30 minutes. Cool slightly to
serve.

Gluten-Free Cranberry Bread

Yields Provided: 12 Servings

Macro Counts For Each Serving:

- Fat Content: 15 g
- Total Net Carbs: 4.7 g
- Protein: 6.4 g
- Calories: 179

What to Use

- Almond flour (2 cups)
- Powdered erythritol or Swerve (.5 cup)
- Steviva stevia powder (.5 tsp.)
- Bak. powder (1.5 tsp.)
- Bak. soda (.5 tsp.)
- Salt (1 tsp.)
- Unsalted butter melted or coconut oil (4 tbsp.)
- Eggs at room temperature (4 large)
- Coconut milk (.5 cup)
- Cranberries (12 oz. bag)
- _Optional_: Blackstrap molasses (1 tsp.)
- Also Needed: 9x5-inch loaf pan

What to Do

1. Program the oven temperature to reach 350° Fahrenheit. Lightly grease the baking pan before you start baking.
2. Sift the flour, baking soda, erythritol or stevia, baking powder, and salt.
3. In another container, combine the eggs, butter, molasses, and coconut milk.
4. Combine it all until well combined.

5. Fold in the rinsed cranberries, and add to the pan.
6. Bake about 1.25 hours. Watch closely when you approach the 1-hour marker since oven temperatures vary.
7. Arrange the pan on a rack to cool (15 min.) before removing from the pan.

<u>Bacon Egg Muffins</u>

Yields Provided: 12 Servings
Macro Counts For Each Serving:
- Fat Content: 23.1 g
- Total Net Carbs: 1 g
- Protein: 21.5 g
- Calories: 301

What to Use
- Bacon (12 slices)
- Large eggs (12)
- Cheddar cheese (8 oz. grated)

What to Do
1. Heat the oven to reach 400° Fahrenheit.
2. Arrange the bacon on wire racks over a rimmed baking pan.
3. Bake for 10 to 12 minutes, removing before it's crispy.
4. Line each tin with bacon.
5. Whisk the eggs and stir in grated cheese and portion into the tin.
6. Lower the oven setting to 350° Fahrenheit. Bake for about 25 minutes until the eggs are set.
7. Transfer the muffins out of the tins and serve warm.

Banana Muffins

Yields Provided: 6 Servings
Macro Counts For Each Serving:
- Fat Content: 30 g
- Total Net Carbs: 4 g
- Protein: 8 g
- Calories: 332

What to Use
- Large eggs (3)
- Coconut oil (.25 cup)
- Monk fruit - 30% extract (.25 tsp.)
- Stevia powder extract (.25 tsp.)
- Vanilla extract (1 tsp.)
- Banana extract (2 tsp.)
- Bak. powder (1 tsp.)
- Coconut flour (.25 cup)
- Almond flour (.75 cup)
- Salt (.25 tsp.)
- Cinnamon (.5 tsp.)
- Mashed avocado (1 medium)
- Pecans (.5 cup chopped)
- *Also Needed*: 6-count muffin tin

What to Do
1. Leave the eggs out to become room temperature.
2. Warm up the oven to 350° Fahrenheit.
3. Generously grease the muffin tin.
4. Whisk the coconut oil with stevia and monk fruit.

5. Whisk in the eggs, vanilla, and banana extracts.
6. In another container, whisk or sift the coconut flour, baking powder, salt, cinnamon, and almond flour.
7. Blend into the coconut oil mixture and the mashed avocado.
8. Fold in the nuts, reserving two tablespoons to sprinkle on top.
9. Empty the batter into the molds and garnish with the nuts.
10. Bake for approximately 25 to 30 minutes.

Breakfast Pizza Waffles

Yields Provided: 2 Servings
Macro Counts For Each Serving:
- Fat Content: 48 g
- Total Net Carbs: 7.6 g
- Protein: 30.7g
- Calories: 604

What to Use
- Large eggs (4)
- Grated parmesan cheese (4 tbsp.)
- Italian seasoning (1 tsp.)
- Psyllium husk powder (1 tbsp.)
- Almond flour (3 tbsp.)
- Baking powder (1 tsp.)
- Salt and pepper (as desired)
- Bacon grease (1 tbsp.)
- Tomato sauce (.5 cup)
- Cheddar cheese (3 oz.)
- _Optional_: Pepperoni (14 slices)

What to Do
1. Prepare using an immersion blender to mix all of the fixings until it thickens (omit the tomato sauce and cheese).
2. Heat the waffle iron. Prepare the batter in two batches.
3. Add the tomato sauce (.25 cup each) and cheese (1.5 oz. each) onto each waffle.
4. Broil for three to five minutes in the oven. Add pepperoni as desired but add the carbs.

Chapter 7: Lunch Recipes

Keto Meatballs

Yields Provided: 6 Servings
Macro Counts For Each Serving:
- Protein: 18 grams
- Net Carbs: 4.2 grams
- Fats: 21.8 grams
- Calories: 301

What to Use
- Salt (as desired)
- Pepper (as desired)
- Coconut oil (2 T)
- Tomato sauce (14 oz.)
- Oregano (1 tsp.)
- Flaxseed meal (1 T)
- Parmesan cheese (2 T)
- Egg (1)
- Ground beef (1.5 lbs.)

What to Do
1. In a mixing bowl, combine the seasoning, oregano, flaxseed, parmesan cheese, egg, and ground beef and mix well.
2. Form the results into 6 equally-sized balls.
3. Add the oil to a pan before placing the pan on the stove over a burner turned to

medium heat. Add in the meatballs and let them brown completely, which should take about 5 minutes per side.

4. Once the meatballs have finished browning, add in the tomato sauce, and let it come to a boil. Once it does, reduce the heat and let everything simmer, covered for approximately 25 minutes.

Pork Rind Bread

Yields Provided: 12 Servings
Macro Counts For Each Serving:
- Fat Content: 13 g
- Total Net Carbs: 1.9 g
- Protein: 9 g
- Calories: 166

What to Use
- Cream cheese (8 oz.)
- Grated mozzarella cheese (2 cups)
- Large eggs (3)
- Grated parmesan cheese (.25 cup)
- Crushed pork rinds (1 cup)
- Baking powder (1 tbsp.)
- Herbs and spices (as desired)
- *Also Needed*: Loaf pan - 5 by 9-inch

What to Do
1. Set the oven temperature to reach 375º Fahrenheit.
2. Prepare a baking tin with the paper.
3. Place both types of cheese into a safe dish. Microwave using the high-power setting for one minute. Stir and microwave for another minute.
4. Fold in the egg with the parmesan, baking powder, and pork rinds. Stir until all ingredients have been incorporated. Spread onto the pan.
5. Bake for 15 to 20 minutes. When ready, add the pan to a cooling rack for about 15

minutes.

Salad with Thai Beef

Yields Provided: 4 Servings
Macro Counts For Each Serving:
- Protein: 21 grams
- Net Carbs: 6.4 grams
- Fats: 23 grams
- Calories: 291

What to Use
- Salt (as desired)
- Pepper (as desired)
- Coconut oil (2 T)
- Arugula (1 c)
- Peanuts (.25 c)
- Jalapeno (.5 minced)
- Cucumber (1 small, peeled, sliced)
- Carrot (.25 c shredded)
- Flank steak (1 lb.)
- Mint (.25 c)
- Sugar (2 T)
- Fish sauce (2 T)

What to Do
1. Start by making sure your oven is heated to 400F.
2. In a small bowl, combine half of the mint, the sugar, fish sauce, and lime juice and mix well. At 2 T of the mixture to the steak and coat well.
3. Broil the steak for approximately 5 minutes per side until it reaches your

desired level of doneness. Let it stand for
5 minutes prior to slicing thinly.

4. In a salad bowl, toss all of the ingredients,
    save the arugula.

5. Plate .25 of the arugula on every plate
    before topping with salad, steak, and
    dressing.

Savory Stuffed Bread

Yields Provided: 10 Servings
Macro Counts For Each Serving:
- Fat Content: 20 g
- Total Net Carbs: 2 g
- Protein: 6 g
- Calories: 202

What to Use
- Baking powder (1.5 tsp.)
- Parsley seasoning (2 tbsp.)
- Sage (1 tsp.)
- Rosemary (1 tsp.)
- Medium eggs (8)
- Cream cheese (1 cup)
- Butter (.5 cup)
- Almond flour (2.5 cups)
- Coconut flour (.25 cup)

What to Do
1. Warm the oven to reach 350° Fahrenheit. Grease a loaf pan.
2. Cream/smash the butter and cream cheese. Fold in the seasonings (parsley, sage, and rosemary).
3. Whisk and break in the egg to form the batter until it's smooth.
4. Combine the almond and coconut flour with the baking powder.
5. Mix all of the fixings until well incorporated.
6. Scoop into the loaf pan.

7. Set the timer and bake for 50 minutes.
    Serve and enjoy.

Salmon and Avocado

Yields Provided: 4 Servings
Macro Counts For Each Serving:
- Protein: 28 grams
- Net Carbs: 5.2 grams
- Fats: 30 grams
- Calories: 373

What to Use
- Salt (as desired)
- Pepper (as desired)
- Coconut oil (2 T)
- Avocado tzatziki (2 c)
- Oregano (1 tsp.)
- Garlic (1 clove grated)
- Yogurt (1 T)
- Lemon zest (1 tsp.)
- Lemon juice (2 T)
- Salmon (24 oz., 4 portions)

What to Do
1. Mix together the pepper, salt, oregano, garlic, yogurt, lemon zest, lemon juice, and oil and combine thoroughly before using the marinade to thoroughly coat the salmon.
2. Let the fish marinate for at least 30 minutes before adding it to a baking dish.
3. Ensure your oven is heated to 400F.
4. Place the fish in the oven and let it cook for about 10 minutes or until it begins to flake easily.

5. Top with avocado tzatziki prior to serving.

Bacon & Cheese Drop Biscuits

Yields Provided: 10 Servings
Macro Counts For Each Serving:
- Fat Content: 14 g
- Total Net Carbs: 2 g
- Protein: 6 g
- Calories: 154

What to Use
- Almond Flour (1.5 cups)
- Onion powder (1 tsp.)
- Bak. powder (1 tbsp.)
- Bak. soda (.5 tsp.)
- Dried parsley (1 tbsp.)
- Garlic salt (1 tsp.)
- Bacon (4 slices)
- Eggs (2)
- Sour cream (.5 cup)
- Bacon grease melted (1 tbsp.)
- Shredded cheddar cheese (.33 cup)
- Shredded smoky bacon cheddar cheese (.33 cup)
- Melted grass-fed butter (3 tbsp.)
- Swerve confectioners or powdered erythritol (.5 tsp.)

What to Do
1. Set the oven temperature in advance to 425° Fahrenheit.
2. Prepare a baking pan with a layer of baking paper.
3. Cook and crumble the bacon.

4. Add the baking powder, almond flour,
    onion powder, garlic salt, and baking soda
    into a mixing container using a fork or
    whisk.
5. Combine the eggs, melted butter, bacon
    grease, bacon, parsley, sour cream.
6. Fold the cheese and combine everything.
7. Scoop the biscuit mixture onto the
    prepared pan.
8. Bake for 11 to 15 minutes. Serve when
    they are like you like them.

Keto Sausage Biscuits
Yields Provided: 6 Servings
Macro Counts For Each Serving:
- Fat Content: 20 g
- Total Net Carbs: 2 g
- Protein: 12 g
- Calories: 250

What to Use
- Cream cheese (2 oz.)
- Mozzarella (2 cups - shredded)
- Eggs (2)
- Almond flour (1 cup)
- Salt & pepper (1 pinch of each)
- Colby jack cheese/another favorite (2 oz.)
- Pre-cooked breakfast sausage patties (6)

What to Do
1. Warm the oven to reach 400° Fahrenheit. Prepare a muffin tin with a spritz of cooking oil.
2. Thinly slice the Colby jack into chunks or squares into a microwave-safe container, adding the mozzarella and cream cheese. Cook at 30-second intervals until softened and melted.
3. Whisk the egg and almond flour. Combine with the cheese mixture.
4. Place on a layer of plastic wrap, and pop into the fridge until firm.
5. Slice into six 3-inch balls. Flatten the balls, place the sausage on the dough,

sliced cheese, and wrap the dough around.

6. Arrange in the muffin tin.
7. Bake until set or for 10 to 15 minutes. Top with additional cheese as desired.

Chapter 8: Dinner Recipes

Pizza Bagels

Yields Provided: 6 Servings
Macro Counts For Each Serving:
- Fat Content: 35 g
- Total Net Carbs: 6 g
- Protein: 28 g
- Calories: 449

What to Use
- Baking powder (1 tbsp.)
- Almond flour (2 cups)
- Garlic powder (1 tsp.)
- Dried Italian seasoning (1 tsp.)
- Onion powder (1 tsp.)
- Large eggs (2 whisked)
- Shredded mozzarella cheese - low moisture (3 cups)
- Cream cheese (3 tbsp.)
- Low-carb pizza sauce (.25 cup)
- Chopped pepperoni slices (2.5 oz.)
- Dried oregano (1 tsp.)
- Shredded parmesan cheese (2 tbsp.)

What to Do
1. Set the oven temperature to reach 425° Fahrenheit. Cover a rimmed baking sheet

with a layer of parchment baking paper or a Silpat.
2. Sift to combine the almond flour, garlic powder, baking powder, dried Italian seasoning, and onion powder.
3. In a large microwave-safe mixing container, combine the mozzarella cheese and cream cheese. Cook for 1.5 minutes. Remove from microwave and stir to combine. Continue heating at 30-second increments as needed.
4. In a mixing bowl, add the eggs and almond flour mixture, mixing until all of the fixings are well incorporated.
5. Once everything is well combined, mix in the pepperoni to the dough. Little by little, add and mix in the sauce. The dough will be fairly soft.
6. Divide the dough into six portions, rolling into a ball.
7. Form a ring. Stretch the ring to make a small hole in the center to form it into a bagel shape.
8. Top each bagel with oregano and parmesan
9. Bake on the middle rack until golden brown or for 12 to 14 minutes.

Shrimp Alfredo

Yields Provided: 4 Servings
Macro Counts For Each Serving:
- Protein: 13 grams
- Net Carbs: 3 grams
- Fats: 20 grams
- Calories: 250

What to Use - Alfredo
- Salt (as desired)
- Pepper (as desired)
- Coconut oil (2 T)
- Garlic powder (.25 tsp.)
- Parmesan cheese (.25 c grated)
- Heavy whipping cream (.25 c)
- Cream cheese (2 oz.)

What to Use – Shrimp
- Coconut oil (2 T + divided)
- Cayenne pepper (.5 tsp.)
- Salt (.5 tsp.)
- Pepper (1 T)
- Onion powder (1 T)
- Garlic powder (1 T)
- Paprika (2 T)
- Shrimp (1 lb.)
- Miracle Noodles (2 packages Fettuccine Style)

What to Do
1. Add the oil and cream cheese to a saucepan before placing the pan on the

stove over a burner turned to low heat. Mix in the parmesan cheese and the heavy whipping cream and mix well before seasoning with pepper, salt, and garlic powder.

2. Ensure the zero carb noodles are dry before placing them in a separate pan, along with 1 T coconut oil, and placing the pan on the stove over a burner turned to medium heat and let them warm for 5 minutes.
3. Add the shrimp and seasonings to a mixing bowl and ensure the shrimp is well seasoned.
4. Add the last of the coconut oil to the skillet before turning up the heat to high and add in the shrimp. Allow the shrimp to cook until the tops have blackened.
5. Top with alfredo sauce prior to serving.

Almond Flour Pizza Crust &
Topping

Yields Provided: 4 Servings - 2 Slices each
Macro Counts For Each Serving:

- Fat Content: 37 g
- Total Net Carbs: 8 g
- Protein: 24 g
- Calories: 466

What to Use

- Blanched almond flour (2 cups)
- Kosher salt - not table salt (1 tsp.)
- Bak. soda (1 tsp.)
- Garlic powder (1 tsp.)
- Large egg (1)

The Topping

- Rao's pizza sauce or keto-friendly option (.5 cup)
- Shredded part-skim mozzarella cheese (6 oz. or 1.5 cups)

What to Do

1. Set the oven ahead of time to reach 400° Fahrenheit. Prepare a baking sheet with a layer of parchment baking paper.
2. Whisk the kosher salt, baking soda, almond flour, and garlic powder.
3. Whisk the egg and mix it into the flour mixture. Knead with the dry fixings to prepare into a smooth dough.

4. Transfer the dough into the prepared baking pan. Cover with another sheet of parchment paper and use a rolling pin to roll into a large (¼-inch-thick circle) 10-inch diameter.
5. Bake for 7-8 minutes. Remove the crust from the oven and increase the temperature to broil. Set a rack six inches below flame.
6. Top the crust with the pizza sauce, mozzarella, and other toppings of choice. If needed, you can cover the edges of the crust with strips of foil to prevent them from scorching.
7. Broil the pizza briefly (2-3 min.). Cool and wait for five minutes before serving.

Stuffed flank steak

Yields Provided: 8 Servings - 2 Slices each
Macro Counts For Each Serving:
- Protein: 21 grams
- Net Carbs: 5 grams
- Fats: 29 grams
- Calories: 299

What to Use
- Salt (as desired)
- Pepper (as desired)
- Coconut oil (2 T)
- Walnuts (2 oz. chopped fine)
- Feta cheese (4 oz. crumbled)
- Lemon zest (1 lemon)
- Garlic (3 cloves sliced)
- Onion (4 oz. diced)
- Swiss chard (1 lb. chopped)
- Flank steak (1.5 lbs.)

What to Do
1. Start by making sure your oven is heated to 350F.
2. Place the walnuts on a baking sheet in an even layer and place the baking sheet in the oven for about 10 minutes, or until the walnuts become fragrant and somewhat browned.
3. Add the oil to a pan before placing the pan on the stove over a burner turned to medium heat. Add in the garlic and

onions and let them cook for about 3 minutes or until they begin to soften.

4. Add in as much of the chard as possible and let it cook until it begins to wilt. Switch out the chard as needed until it has all wilted.

5. Place all of the chard in a large mixing bowl before adding in the lemon zest, seasoning as desired, and mixing well.

6. While the chard is cooling, create a trench in the flank steak by cutting into it for most of its length and stopping about .5 inches from the other side. Once you complete both sides, you should be able to open each steak as if it were a book.

7. Add oil to the steak before mixing together the salt and pepper and using the results to season as desired.

8. Mix the remaining ingredients into the chard and add the results to each steak. Tie the steak together using kitchen twine as needed.

9. Heat your grill to a high/medium heat before placing the steak on the grill and grilling until the steak's internal temperature reaches 160 degrees.

10. Let the steak rest for 10 minutes prior to serving.

Chicken Crust Pizza

Yields Provided: 8 Servings
Macro Counts For Each Serving:
- Fat Content: 13 g
- Total Net Carbs: 0.8 g
- Protein: 14 g
- Calories: 172

What to Use
- Chicken thighs (1 lb.)
- Shredded mozzarella - whole milk (1 cup)
- Large egg (1)
- Dried oregano (1 tsp.)
- Black pepper and salt (.25 tsp. each)
- Butter (2 tbsp.)
- Celery (1 stalk)
- Sour cream (1 tbsp.)
- Franks Red Hot Original (3 tbsp.)
- Blue cheese crumbles (1 oz.)
- Green onion (1 stalk)

What to Do

1. Set the oven temperature to 400°
   Fahrenheit. Cut and place a sheet of
   parchment paper onto a pizza pan and
   set aside.
2. Remove all of the bones and skin from
   the chicken. Grind using the blade
   attachment on a food processor into a
   large mixing container. Finely dice the
   celery.
3. Whisk and add the egg, salt, and .5 cup
   of shredded mozzarella to the mixing
   container.
4. Mix the crust until all of the shredded
   cheese is enclosed in the dough.
5. Spread the chicken out until it's .25-inch
   thick in the pizza pan. Bake until the
   crust is starting to brown on top (25
   min.).
6. Meanwhile, add and melt the butter in a
   skillet and sauté the celery until it wilts.
7. Blend in 2 tbsp. of hot sauce and sour
   cream.
8. Remove the crust and add the sauce
   layered with the celery, rest of the
   mozzarella, and crumbles of blue cheese.
9. Bake until the cheese is melted (10 min.).
   Switch to broil for the last few minutes.
10. Drizzle hot sauce and garnish with green
    onion slices before serving.

Biscuits & Gravy

Yields Provided: 2 Servings
Macro Counts For Each Serving:
- Fat Content: 60 g
- Total Net Carbs: 3 g
- Protein: 40 g
- Calories: 737

What to Use
Cheddar Biscuits
- Melted butter (.25 cup)
- Eggs (4 large)
- Coconut flour (.33 cup)
- Salt (.25 tsp.)
- Bak. powder (.25 tsp.)
- Shredded cheddar cheese (1 cup)

Gravy
- Chicken broth (1 cup)
- Ground sausage (1 lb.)
- Heavy cream (1 cup)
- Xanthan gum (.5 tsp.)
- Black pepper & salt (as desired)

What to Do
1. Warm the oven in advance to reach 400° Fahrenheit.
2. Prepare a baking pan with a layer of parchment baking paper or spritz using a cooking oil spray.
3. Combine the biscuit fixings in a large bowl. Stir to combine.

4. Scoop 3 tbsp. worth of batter for each biscuit.
5. Arrange them two inches apart on the baking tin.
6. Bake for approximately 15 minutes. Transfer to the countertop.
7. Brown and crumble the sausage using the med-high heat setting until it is cooked through.
8. Pour in the chicken broth, xanthan gum, salt, pepper, and cream. Stir to combine.
9. Bring it to a simmer. Lower the heat and continue simmering until the gravy is thick. Remove from the burner.
10. Slice the biscuits in half and spoon gravy over the biscuits.

<u>Cheeseburger Casserole</u>

Yields Provided: 6 Servings
Macro Counts For Each Serving:
- Protein: 32 grams
- Net Carbs: 6 grams
- Fats: 53 grams
- Calories: 628

What to Use
- Salt (as desired)
- Pepper (as desired)
- Coconut oil (2 T)
- Dill (1 tsp.)
- Cheddar cheese (8 oz. shredded)
- Hot sauce (1 tsp.)
- Heavy cream (.25 c)
- Eggs (4 large)
- Worcestershire sauce (1 T)
- Yellow mustard (1 T)
- Ketchup (2 T)
- Cream cheese (4 T)
- Garlic (1 clove)
- Onion (.5)
- Ground beef (1 lb.)
- Bacon (.5 lbs.)

What to Do
1. Start by making sure your oven is heated to 350F.
2. Add the oil to a pan before placing the pan on the stove over a burner turned to medium heat.

3. Dice the bacon and add it to the skillet, stirring regularly until it is crisp. Remove the bacon from the skillet but retain the grease.
4. Add in the garlic along with the beef and onion and allow it all to cook for approximately 5 minutes. Mix in the seasonings, Worcestershire sauce, mustard, ketchup, and cream cheese and combine thoroughly.
5. Add the results to a prepared baking dish (8x8) and then add the bacon on top.
6. Add the eggs to a mixing bowl, add in the heavy cream and mix to combine before seasoning as desired and adding in the hot sauce.
7. Pour the result into the baking dish before topping with the cheddar cheese.
8. Add the baking dish to the oven for 30 minutes. Top with dill prior to serving.

Salmon and Cream Sauce

Yields Provided: 2 Servings
Macro Counts For Each Serving:
- Protein: 28 grams
- Net Carbs: 4 grams
- Fats: 39 grams
- Calories: 431

What to Use
- Salt (as desired)
- Pepper (as desired)
- Coconut oil (2 T)
- Sockeye salmon filets (2, 6 oz.)
- Lemon zest (.5 tsp.)
- Vodka (1 T + .25 c)
- Water (2 T)
- Heavy cream (.3 c)
- Tomato paste (1 T)
- Onion (1 oz. sliced)
- Garlic (1 clove)
- Bacon (2 slices diced)

What to Do
1. Set the salmon out on the counter and let it reach room temperature as you prepare the other ingredients
2. Place a medium-sized frying pan over medium heat. Add the bacon and 1 teaspoon of bacon grease and stir, coating the bacon. Let cook about 2 minutes. Meanwhile, slice the onion and garlic, chiffonade the basil, and grate the lemon

zest. (To chiffonade, stack the basil leaves, roll them lengthwise, then cutting crosswise, slice into thin ribbons.) Give the bacon in the pan a stir and cook until browned and crisp. Remove the bacon leaving the fat in the pan.

3. Turn the burner to medium heat and lightly salt the salmon before adding it to the pan with the skin facing up. Let it cook for about 3 minutes per side.
4. Plate the fish before covering it with foil to keep it warm.
5. Reduce the heat on the pan slightly before adding in the garlic and onion and cooking for 90 seconds.
6. Remove the pan from the oven and carefully and slowly add in the vodka, this can cause injury if you are not careful, so caution is recommended.
7. Place the pan back on the stove and stir well until the vodka reduces 50 percent.
8. Add in the tomato paste and stir well before adding in the water and heavy cream and combining thoroughly. Allow it to simmer for 60 seconds before adding in the bacon, lemon zest, and remaining vodka. Season as desired and stir until the smell of alcohol evaporates.
9. Top the salmon with the sauce prior to serving

Crunchy Cheese Pizza

Yields Provided: 4 Servings (2 slices each)
Macro Counts For Each Serving:

- Fat Content: 23 g
- Total Net Carbs: 1 g
- Protein: 19 g
- Calories: 298

What to Use

- Pepperoni (2 oz.)
- Mushrooms (3)
- Oregano (2 pinch - dried)
- Keto-friendly marinara sauce (2 tbsp.)
- Shredded cheddar cheese (.5 cup)
- Shredded mozzarella cheese (2 cups)
- _Also Needed:_ High-heat non-stick skillet

What to Do

1. Thinly slice the pepperoni and
    mushrooms and toss onto a lined cookie
    sheet. Broil/grill for 3 to 5 minutes.
2. Place the pan using the high-heat
    temperature setting. Spread the
    mozzarella cheese evenly over the pan,
    then sprinkle over the cheddar. Work the
    cheese in off the edges of the pan.
    Sprinkle over the oregano.
3. Spread the marinara sauce around the
    melting cheese, try not to work it down
    into the cheese rather over it.
4. Add the pepperoni and mushrooms.
5. When the base is golden brown, crispy,
    and begins to lift as one piece, your pizza
    is ready.
6. Carefully slide the pizza off onto a
    chopping board or cutting surface and cut
    into 8 equal pieces.
7. Serve.

Yellow-Fin Tuna with Poke

Yields Provided: 2 Servings
Macro Counts For Each Serving:
- Protein: 29 grams
- Net Carbs: 4.8 grams
- Fats: 33 grams
- Calories: 445

What to Use
- Salt (as desired)
- Pepper (as desired)
- Red grapefruit (.25)
- Pili nuts (.25 c)
- Sesame seeds (1 T)
- Sesame oil (2 T)
- Avocado (.5)
- Cilantro (5 sprigs)
- Coconut aminos (1 T)
- Ahi tuna (8 oz.)

What to Do
1. Slice the tuna into .25 in. cubes and add to a large mixing bowl before mixing in the salt, pepper, sesame oil and coconut aminos and toss gently.
2. Add in the grapefruit, pili nuts, avocado, and cilantro and mix well.
3. Divide the results into two bowls, and top with sesame seeds prior to serving.

Chorizo with Scallops

Yields Provided: 4 Servings
Macro Counts For Each Serving:
- Protein: 30 grams
- Net Carbs: 2 grams
- Fats: 33.7 grams
- Calories: 469

What to Use
- Salt (as desired)
- Pepper (as desired)
- Lemon juice (2 T)
- Parsley (4 T chopped)
- Parmesan cheese (1 c grated)
- Heavy whipping cream (.25 c)
- Chorizo (4.2 oz.)
- Spinach (2 lbs. frozen)
- Coconut oil (2 T)
- Scallops (1 lb.)

What to Do
1. Add the oil to a pan before placing the pan on the stove over a burner turned to a high/medium heat. Let the chorizo cook for approximately 5 minutes, and it is nice and crispy. Once it has cooked, remove the chorizo from the bowl but retain the grease.
2. Clean the scallops and season them as desired before adding them to the pan and cooking for 2 minutes per side. If the

scallop sticks to the pan, the side needs a little more time.

3. After the scallops are cooked, return the chorizo to the pan and heat it for an additional 60 seconds. Remove the scallops and chorizo from the pan and plate.
4. Add 2 T more oil to the pan before adding in the garlic and spinach and cook for 2 minutes before adding in the cream and the cheese and mixing well. Let everything cook and additional 2 minutes.
5. Add the spinach to the top of the scallops and chorizo prior to serving.

Feta & Spinach Dinner Muffins

Yields Provided: 6 Servings
Macro Counts For Each Serving:
- Fat Content: 16 g
- Total Net Carbs: 2 g
- Protein: 14 g
- Calories: 208

What to Use
- Eggs (6)
- Bacon (3 slices - cooked)
- Raw spinach (2 cups)
- Crumbled feta cheese (1 cup)
- Cheddar cheese (.5 cup)
- Black pepper & salt (as desired)

What to Do
1. Warm the oven in advance to reach 350° Fahrenheit.
2. Rinse the spinach under cold water. Drain and toss into a microwave-safe container. Cook on high for one minute. Set aside for a few minutes.
3. In another mixing container, whisk the eggs until frothy.
4. Fold in grated cheddar cheese, crumbled feta cheese, and bacon pieces.
5. Once the spinach is cooled enough, add to the bowl, and mix until combined. Divide into the six muffin cups.
6. Bake for 30-35 minutes until muffins are firm.

Keto Pizza with a Low-Carb Broccoli Pizza Crust

Yields Provided: 4 Servings
Macro Counts For Each Serving:
- Fat Content: g
- Total Net Carbs: g
- Protein: g
- Calories: 115

What to Use
- Broccoli rice (two 12 oz. bags) frozen—thawed or fresh (3 cups)
- Large egg (1)
- Freshly grated parmesan cheese (.66 cup)
- Optional: Super-fine blanched almond flour, optional but helped to give the crust a crispier texture (2 tbsp.)
- Garlic powder (.5 tsp.)
- Dried oregano (1 tsp.) optional
- Dried basil (.5 tsp.) optional

Toppings
- Grated mozzarella (.33 cup)
- Sugar-free marinara sauce (Rao's) or passata sauce (.25 cup)
- Pepperoni (6-8 slices)
- Sliced mushrooms (.25 cup)
- Fresh basil or spinach (3-4 leaves)
- Chopped olives (2-3)

What to Do

1. Warm the oven in advance to reach 425°
    Fahrenheit.
2. Arrange the frozen broccoli rice in a
    microwavable dish and cook using high
    for three to five minutes. Or, place it in
    the oven for 10 minutes, rotating the pan
    and cool for about ten minutes.
3. Combine the prepared broccoli flour, egg,
    mozzarella, and optional seasonings.
    Knead well to form the dough.
4. Cover the baking sheet with a layer of
    parchment baking paper. Add the dough
    and roll out using a rolling pin to reach
    about .25 to .5-inch thickness.
5. Make a raised edge and bake for 15
    minutes.
6. Remove and add the sauce and desired
    toppings.
7. Top it off using the mozzarella and bake
    until the cheese has melted. Slice and
    serve while piping hot.

Chapter 9: Snack Recipes

Jicama Chips

Yields Provided: 6 Servings
Macro Counts For Each Serving:
- Protein: 1.2 grams
- Net Carbs: 4 grams
- Fats: 8 grams
- Calories: 38

What to Use
- Salt (as desired)
- Pepper (as desired)
- Coconut oil (2 T)

What to Do
1. Start by making sure your oven is heated to 400F.
2. Prepare a baking sheet by lining it with parchment paper
3. Add the oil to a pan before placing the pan on the stove over a burner turned to medium heat. Slice the jicama into thin strips and let them cook long enough to absorb the oil.
4. Place the chips onto the baking sheet in a single layer so that they do not overlap before seasoning as desired.
5. Place the baking sheet in the oven for 20 minutes or until the chips are crisp.

6. Let cool 10 minutes prior to serving.

Sesame Seed Bread

Yields Provided: 6 Servings
Macro Counts For Each Serving:
- Fat Content: 13 g
- Total Net Carbs: 1 g
- Protein: 7 g
- Calories: 100

What to Use
- Boiling water (1 cup)
- Almond flour (1.25 cups)
- Bak. powder (2 tsp.)
- Sesame seeds (2 tbsp.)
- Psyllium husk powder (5 tbsp.)
- Sea salt (.25 tsp.)
- Apple cider vinegar (2 tsp.)
- Egg whites (3)

What to Do
1. Set the oven temperature to reach 350° Fahrenheit.
2. Spritz a baking sheet with cooking oil spray. Put the water in a saucepan to boil.
3. Mix the sea salt, baking powder, almond flour, sesame seeds, and psyllium powder.
4. Stir in hot water, vinegar, and egg whites. Use a hand mixer (less than 1 min.) to combine. Place the bread on the prepared pan.
5. Bake for one hour on the lowest oven rack. Serve and enjoy any time.

Keto Bread

Yields Provided: 6 Servings
Macro Counts For Each Serving:
- Protein: 28 grams
- Net Carbs: 2.7 grams
- Fats: 30 grams
- Calories: 273

What to Use
- Water (2 c boiling)
- Eggs (2 large)
- Egg whites (6 large)
- Sea salt (1 T)
- Baking powder (1 T)
- Sesame seed flour (.75 c)
- Coconut flour (.5 c)
- Psyllium husk powder (.3 c)
- Almond flour (1 c)

What to Do
1. Start by making sure your oven is heated to 350F.
2. Prepare a loaf pan by lining it with parchment paper, take care to ensure you leave some to hang over the edges.
3. Add the egg whites and eggs to a mixing bowl and mix well before setting them aside.
4. Add all of the dry ingredients to a separate mixing bowl and combine thoroughly before adding in the eggs and mixing well using a mixer.

5. Add to the loaf pan before placing it in the oven and letting it bake for 75 minutes.
6. Allow the bread to cool fully prior to slicing.

Zucchini Chips

Yields Provided: 2 Servings
Macro Counts For Each Serving:
- Protein: 2 grams
- Net Carbs: 5 grams
- Fats: 10 grams
- Calories: 100

What to Use
- Salt (as desired)
- Pepper (as desired)
- Coconut oil (2 T)
- Garlic powder (.25 tsp.)
- Curry powder (.25 tsp.)
- Zucchini (2)

What to Do
1. Start by making sure your oven is heated to 225F.
2. Prepare 2 baking sheets by lining them with parchment paper.
3. Cut the ends of the zucchini off and discard. Very thinly slice the zucchini into paper thin rounds.
4. Place the zucchini rounds in a single layer on the prepared parchment-lined baking sheets. Place them close together, but don't let the zucchini rounds touch each other.
5. Brush the tops of the zucchini with oil.

6. Combine the curry powder, garlic powder, and salt in a small bowl and sprinkle evenly over oil-coated zucchini slices.
7. Bake for 60 minutes or until the zucchini becomes crisp.
8. When the chips have cooled, store in an airtight container.

<u>*Onion Crackers with Thyme*</u>

Yields Provided: 15Servings
Macro Counts For Each Serving:
- Protein: 2.7 grams
- Net Carbs: .7 grams
- Fats: 8 grams
- Calories: 88

What to Use
- Salt (as desired)
- Pepper (as desired)
- Sunflower seeds (.25 c finely ground)
- Flax seeds (1.5 c)
- Thyme (2 tsp.)
- Avocado oil (.25 c)
- Garlic (1 clove minced)
- Onion (1 c chopped)

What to Do
1. Start by making sure your oven is heated to 225F.
2. Add the pepper, salt, thyme, oil, garlic, and onion to a food processor and process vigorously. Add in the seeds and pulse enough to combine the ingredients.
3. Add the results to a large bowl. Using a 10-inch piece of parchment paper, scoop out about .5 c of the dough and roll it into a ball. Fold the parchment paper around the ball and then use it to roll the dough flat until it is about .25 inches thick. Rip off the top of the parchment paper and

score the dough into 1-inch squares. Place the parchment paper on the baking sheet and repeat as needed.

4. Place the baking sheet in the oven for 2 hours, flip halfway through the process, and remove the last of the parchment paper. Baking time may vary based on the thickness of the crackers.
5. Let cool for 15 minutes prior to serving.

Macadamia Nut Hummus

Yields Provided: 8 Servings
Macro Counts For Each Serving:
- Protein: 1.7 grams
- Net Carbs: 2.8 grams
- Fats: 17 grams
- Calories: 116

What to Use
- Salt (as desired)
- Pepper (as desired)
- Coconut oil (2 T)
- Cayenne pepper (1 pinch)
- Tahini (2 T)
- Water (3 T)
- Lemon juice (3 T)
- Garlic (2 cloves)
- Macadamia nuts (1 c soaked in water for 24 hours, drained, rinsed)

What to Do
1. Add all of the ingredients to your food processor and process until smooth.
2. Serve promptly for best results.

Radish Chips

Yields Provided: 4 Servings
Macro Counts For Each Serving:
- Protein: 1.1 grams
- Net Carbs: 2.4 grams
- Fats: 9.7 grams
- Calories: 48

What to Use
- Salt (as desired)
- Pepper (as desired)
- Coconut oil (.5 c)
- Radishes (16 oz.)

What to Do
1. Add the oil to a deep saucepan before placing it on the stove over a burner turned to medium heat.
2. Slice the radishes using an extremely sharp knife to ensure the slices are as thin as possible.
3. Add the radishes to a pot before covering them with water, and placing the pot on the stove over a burner turned to high heat. Let them boil for 5 minutes, and they have turned nearly translucent.
4. Drain the radishes before adding them slowly to the hot oil to ensure there is no splatter.
5. Let the radishes fry for approximately 8 minutes or until they have turned a deep, golden brown.

6. Drain, season as desired and let cool prior
    to serving

Herb Crackers

Yields Provided: 15 Servings
Macro Counts For Each Serving:
- Protein: 4.4 grams
- Net Carbs: .9 grams
- Fats: 10.8 grams
- Calories: 185

What to Use
- Salt (as desired)
- Pepper (as desired)
- Coconut oil (2 T)
- Rosemary (5 g)
- Thyme (5 g)
- Apple cider vinegar (2)
- Avocado oil (.25 c)
- Celery (10 sticks)
- Flaxseed (3 c ground roughly)

What to Do
1. Start by making sure your oven is heated to 225F.
2. Add the pepper, salt, herbs, vinegar, oil, and celery into a food processor and process vigorously. Add in the seeds and pulse enough to combine the ingredients. All the results to sit for 2 minutes to firm.
3. Add the results to a large bowl. Using a 10-inch piece of parchment paper, scoop out about .5 c of the dough and roll it into a ball. Fold the parchment paper around the ball and then use it to roll the dough

flat until it is about .25 inches thick. Rip off the top of the parchment paper and score the dough into 1-inch squares. Place the parchment paper on the baking sheet and repeat as needed.

4. Place the baking sheet in the oven for 2 hours, flip halfway through the process, and remove the last of the parchment paper. Baking time may vary based on the thickness of the crackers.

5. Let cool for 15 minutes prior to serving.

Onion Soup Mix

Yields Provided: 4 Servings
Macro Counts For Each Serving:
- Protein: 1 gram
- Net Carbs: 1.9 grams
- Fats: 4 grams
- Calories: 27

What to Use
- Salt (as desired)
- Pepper (as desired)
- Herbamare (.5 tsp.)
- Celery salt (1 tsp.)
- Turmeric (2 tsp.)
- Onion powder (2 tsp.)
- Parsley flakes (1 T)
- Onion (.6 c minced

What to Do
1. Combine all the ingredients together in a mason jar and mix well.

Chapter 10: Dessert Recipes

Keto Cheesecake Bites

Yields Provided: 9 Servings
Macro Counts For Each Serving:
- Protein: 5 grams
- Net Carbs: 1 gram
- Fats: 29 grams
- Calories: 286

What to Use
Cheesecake
- Swerve (.3 c)
- Caramel syrup (1 T sugar-free)
- Espresso (3 T)
- Eggs (3)
- Unsalted butter (2 T)
- Cream cheese (8 oz. softened)

Frosting
- Mascarpone cheese (8 oz. softened)
- Swerve (2 T)
- Caramel syrup (3 T sugar-free)
- Unsalted butter (3 T softened)

What to Do
1. Start by making sure your oven is heated to 350F.

2. Prepare a cupcake tin and line it with cupcake liners.
3. Combine all of the ingredients for the cheesecake in a blender and blend well. Pour the results into the cupcake tin.
4. Place the cupcake tin in the oven for 15 minutes. Remove the cheesecake from the oven and place them in the refrigerator to chill for at least 3 hours.
5. To make the frosting, start by creaming the butter before adding it to a mixing bowl along with the swerve and caramel syrup. Add the results to the blender and slowly blend in the mascarpone cheese.
6. Add the frosting to the cheesecake prior to serving.

Lemon Mousse

Yields Provided: 5 Servings
Macro Counts For Each Serving:
- Protein: 3.7 grams
- Net Carbs: 1.7 grams
- Fats: 30 grams
- Calories: 277

What to Use
- Salt (1 pinch)
- Lemon-flavored stevia (.5 tsp.)
- Heavy cream (1 c)
- Lemon juice (.25 c)
- Mascarpone cheese (8 oz.)

What to Do
1. In a standing mixer, blend together the lemon juice and mascarpone cheese until smooth.
2. Add in the remaining ingredients and blend until everything is whipped.
3. Add the results to a piping bag before pipping into serving glasses and place the serving glasses in the refrigerator and allow them to chill.
4. Top with lemon zest prior to serving.

Chocolate Pudding

Yields Provided: 2 Servings
Macro Counts For Each Serving:
- Protein: 1.1 grams
- Net Carbs: .5 grams
- Fats: 10 grams
- Calories: 90

What to Use
- Glucomannan powder (.5 tsp.)
- Dark cocoa powder (1 T)
- Stevia (2 T)
- Coconut milk (1 c)

What to Do
1. In a microwave-safe bowl, combine the coconut milk, cocoa powder, and stevia and whisk thoroughly. Add in the glucomannan powder and whisk well to prevent lumps.
2. Add the bowl to the microwave and heat it on high for 90 seconds.
3. Whisk once more before covering the bowl and letting it chill for at least 2 hours prior to serving.

Pumpkin Bread

Yields Provided: 12 Servings
Macro Counts For Each Serving:
- Fat Content: 18 g
- Total Net Carbs: 4 g
- Protein: 8 g
- Calories: 215

What to Use
- Blanched almond flour (2 cups)
- Coconut flour (.5 cup)
- Erythritol (.75 cup)
- Pumpkin pie spice (2 tsp.)
- Sea salt (.25 tsp.)
- Gluten-free bak. powder (2 tsp.)
- Pumpkin puree (.75 cup)
- Eggs (4 large - lightly beaten)
- Butter (measured solid, then melted; can use ghee or coconut oil (.33 cup)
- Pumpkin seeds (.25 cup)
- _Also Needed_: Loaf pan 9 by 5-inches

What to Do
1. Warm the oven to reach 350° Fahrenheit
2. Prepare the pan with parchment baking paper. Leave some of the bag hanging over the edges for easy removal later.
3. Sift or whisk the coconut flour, erythritol, almond flour, pumpkin pie spice, sea salt, and baking powder.
4. Fold in the pumpkin puree, eggs, and melted butter. Mix well.

5. Empty the batter into the lined pan. Sprinkle the top with pumpkin seeds and press them lightly into the surface.
6. Bake for 50 minutes to one hour.
7. Cool completely before removing from the pan and slicing.

Cookie Bars

Yields Provided: 12 Servings
Macro Counts For Each Serving:
- Protein: 1.2 grams
- Net Carbs: .3 grams
- Fats: 12 grams
- Calories: 143

What to Use
- Coconut oil (.3 c melted +1 T)
- Coconut (2 c shredded)
- Unsweetened chocolate (3 squares)
- Stevia (24 drops divided)

What to Do
1. Add 12 drops of stevia, .3 cups of melted coconut oil, and the shredded coconut to a food processor and process well.
2. Add the results to a silicone loaf pan and place the pan into the freezer so the contents can freeze.
3. Add the chocolate and the remaining coconut oil to a microwavable bowl and place it in the microwave before heating it for 40 seconds on a 50 percent heat.
4. Mix in 12 drops of stevia to the results and stir well.
5. Add the results to the top of the frozen ingredients and freeze for an additional 30 minutes
6. Cut into squares prior to serving.

Raspberry Lemon Popsicle

Yields Provided: 6 Servings
Macro Counts For Each Serving:
- Protein: .5 grams
- Net Carbs: 2 grams
- Fats: 5 grams
- Calories: 150

What to Use
- Lemon (.5 juiced)
- Coconut oil (.25 c)
- Coconut milk (1 c)
- Sour cream (.25 c)
- Heavy cream (.25 c)
- Guar gum (.5 tsp.)
- Stevia (20 drops)
- Raspberries (3.5 oz.)

What to Do
1. Combine all of the ingredients using an immersion blender and strain the results to remove any seeds.
2. Add the results to popsicle molds.
3. Freeze for 2 hours.

Cheesecake smoothie

Yields Provided: 1 Servings
Macro Counts For Each Serving:
- Protein: 6.4 grams
- Net Carbs: 5.2 grams
- Fats: 53 grams
- Calories: 515

What to Use
- Vanilla extract (.5 t)
- Water (.5 c)
- Raspberries (.5 c frozen)
- Coconut oil (1 T)
- Coconut milk (.75 c)
- Stevia (25 drops)

What to Do
1. Cream the coconut milk: This is a simple process. All you need to do is place the can of coconut milk in the refrigerator overnight. The next morning, open the can and spoon out the coconut milk that has solidified. Don't shake the can before opening. Discard the liquids.
2. Add all of the ingredients, save the ice cubes, to the blender, and blend on a low speed until pureed. Thin with water as needed.

Key Lime Smoothie

Yields Provided: 1 Servings
Macro Counts For Each Serving:
- Protein: 10 grams
- Net Carbs: 2.4 grams
- Fats: 22 grams
- Calories: 340

What to Use
- Almond milk (1 c)
- Avocado (.5)
- Lime zest (1 lime)
- Vanilla extract (.5 tsp.)
- Sea salt (1 pinch)
- Stevia (25 drops)

What to Do
1. Add all of the ingredients to a blender and blend until smooth. Take care to add the liquids prior to adding in the solids for the best results.

Black Walnut Chocolate Chip Keto Muffins

Yields Provided: 12 Servings
Macro Counts For Each Serving:
- Fat Content: 26.1 g
- Total Net Carbs: 5.1 g
- Protein: 8.3 g
- Calories: 292

What to Use
- Almond flour (3 cups)
- Firmly packed coconut flour (4 tbsp.)
- Bak. powder (1 tbsp.)
- Bak. soda (1 tsp.)
- Salt (1 tsp.)
- Monk fruit (.75 cup)
- Melted ghee (6 tbsp.)
- Canned coconut milk - Full-fat (6 tbsp.)
- Unchilled large eggs (3)
- Vanilla extract (1 tbsp.)
- Stevia-sweetened chocolate chips (.5 cup + 1 tbsp.)
- Black walnuts (.25 cup - diced)

What to Do
1. Warm the oven to 350° Fahrenheit. Generously spritz a muffin pan with a mist of cooking oil spray.
2. Whisk or sift the almond and coconut flour, salt, baking powder, and baking soda into a mixing container.

3. Using an electric hand mixer, blend the monk fruit, coconut milk, ghee, eggs, and vanilla.
4. Fold in the flour mixture and stir well. Next, fold in the chocolate chips and walnuts. Let the dough rest for about five minutes so the coconut flour can begin to absorb the moisture.
5. Fill the muffin tins about two/thirds of the way to the top.
6. Bake for about 25 to 30 minutes.
7. Cool in the pan. If needed, use a butter knife around each muffin to loosen them for serving.

Brownie Pumpkin Muffins

Yields Provided: 6 Servings
Macro Counts For Each Serving:
- Fat Content: 13 g
- Total Net Carbs: 4.4 g
- Protein: 7 g
- Calories: 183

What to Use
- Salt (.5 tsp.)
- Flaxseed meal (1 cup)
- Cocoa powder (.25 cup)
- Cinnamon (1 tbsp.)
- Baking powder (.5 tbsp.)
- Coconut oil (2 tbsp.)
- Large egg (1)
- Sugar-free caramel syrup (.25 cup)
- Vanilla extract (1 tsp.)
- Pumpkin puree (.5 cup)
- Slivered almonds (.5 cup)
- Apple cider vinegar (1 tsp.)

What to Do
1. Set the oven temperature at 350° Fahrenheit.
2. Combine each of the fixings and stir well.
3. Use six paper liners in the muffin tin, and add .25 cup of batter into each one. Sprinkle several almonds on the tops, pressing gently.
4. Bake approximately 15 minutes or when the top is set.

<u>Chocolate Chip & Peanut Butter Mini Muffins</u>

Yields Provided: 24 Servings
Macro Counts For Each Serving:
- Fat Content: 9.8 g
- Total Net Carbs: 4.3 g
- Protein: 8.1 g
- Calories: 131

What to Use
- Peanut flour (1 cup)
- Salt (.25 tsp.)
- Bak. powder (1.5 tsp.)
- Peanut butter (.33 cup)
- Butter/coconut oil (2 tbsp.)
- Golden low carb sweetener or other brown sugar replacement (.33 cup)
- Large egg (1)
- Almond milk or coconut milk (.33 cup)
- Sugar-free chocolate chips (.25 cup)

What to Do
1. In advance, set the oven temperature to reach 350° Fahrenheit.
2. Prepare the (24- count) mini muffin pan with baking cups.
3. Sift the salt with the peanut flour and baking powder.
4. In another container, mix the peanut butter, butter, and sweetener until creamy.

5. Fold in the whisked egg and milk until smooth.
6. Combine everything until blended.
7. Lastly, add in the chocolate chips.
8. Scoop the batter into the cups using a cookie scoop for convenience.
9. Bake for 10-12 minutes.
10. Set to the side and cool for about five minutes

<u>*Coffee Cake Muffins*</u>

Yields Provided: 12 Servings
Macro Counts For Each Serving:

- Fat Content: 18 g
- Total Net Carbs: 5 g
- Protein: 7 g
- Calories: 222

What to Use
Batter

- Unchilled butter (2 tbsp.)
- Unchilled cream cheese (2 oz.)
- Stevia or favorite sweetener (.33 cup)
- Eggs (4)
- Vanilla (2 tsp.)
- Unsweetened vanilla almond milk (.5 cup)
- Almond flour (1 cup)
- Bak. powder (1 tsp.)
- Coconut flour (.5 cup)
- Salt (.25 tsp.)

Topping

- Almond flour (1 cup)
- Coconut flour (2 tbsp.)
- Stevia/your choice (.25 cup)
- Softened butter (.25 cup)
- Cinnamon (1 tsp.)
- *Optional*: Molasses (.5 tsp.)
- *Also Needed*: Standard muffin tin & Parchment baking paper

What to Do

1. Soften the butter and cream cheese for about 30 minutes on the countertop before preparing the recipe.
2. Warm the oven to reach 350° Fahrenheit.
3. Prepare the tin with a spritz of cooking oil spray.
4. Combine all the batter fixings in a food processor. Mix thoroughly and pour into the muffin tin.
5. Combine the topping fixings in the food processor. Pulse until crumbs form. Sprinkle on top of the batter.
6. Bake 20-25 min until golden.
7. *Note:* If the crumb topping starts to get too dark cover with foil for the last 5 minutes.

Conclusion

Thank you for making it through to the end of *Ketogenic Diet for Beginners: Living the Keto Lifestyle*, let's hope it was informative and able to provide you with all of the tools you need to achieve your weight loss goals, whatever it is that they may be. Just because you've finished this book doesn't mean there is nothing left to learn on the topic, expanding your horizons is the only way to find the success you seek.

I hope this guide has helped you eat healthier and lose weight by achieving ketosis. The ketogenic world is constantly growing, and every day more and more people are discovering this amazing lifestyle.

Because the number of followers of ketogenic way of eating is growing every day, there are plenty of books on the market covering this topic. I am thankful you chose to purchase this one. I hope it gave you all the information you needed to help you better understand the ketogenic diet, understand ketosis, and jump-start your journey to better health through having a body that is fat-fueled rather that sugar-fueled.

Your support is always welcome. If you enjoyed this book and gained new knowledge, please take the time to share your thoughts and post a review on Amazon to help other people live and eat healthier. It would be greatly appreciated!

Thank you again, and good luck with your keto diet experience.

9 781712 548288